SCATTERED LIMBS

Also by Iain Bamforth

A Doctor's Dictionary
The Crossing Fee
The Good European
A Place in the World
The Body in the Library
Open Workings
Sons and Pioneers

SCATTERED LIMBS
A Medical Dreambook

by

Iain Bamforth

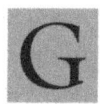

G

Galileo Publishers, Cambridge

Galileo Publishers
16 Woodlands Road
Great Shelford
Cambridge CB22 5LW
UK

www.galileopublishing.co.uk

Distributed in the USA by:
SCB Distributors
15608 S. New Century Drive
Gardena, CA 90248-2129

ISBN 978-1-903385-95-1

First published in the UK 2020

© 2020 Iain Bamforth
© 2020 Galileo Publishers

Illustrations by Claire Bamforth

All rights reserved.
This book is sold subject to the
condition that it shall not, by way of trade or
otherwise, be lent, resold, hired out or otherwise
circulated in any form of binding or cover other than that
in which it is published and without a similar condition
including this condition being imposed
on the subsequent purchaser.

1 2 3 4 5 6 7 8 9
Printed in the EU

In memory of my father-in-law Christian Schütze (1927-2018)

"Truly, my friends, I walk among men as among
the fragments and limbs of men…"

Friedrich Nietzsche, "On Redemption",
Also sprach Zarathustra

"The province of Medicine seems… to constitute
a kind of Alsatia, an enclave in the Universe, of which the
exploitation is permitted to the licensed few."

F. G. Crookshank, "The Importance of a Theory of Signs
and a Critique of Language in the Study of Medicine",
in Ogden's *The Meaning of Meaning*

"I've gone from nation to nation to learn my trade
And now I've come back to Scotland to cure the dead."

Abbotsford version of the mummers play *Galoshins*

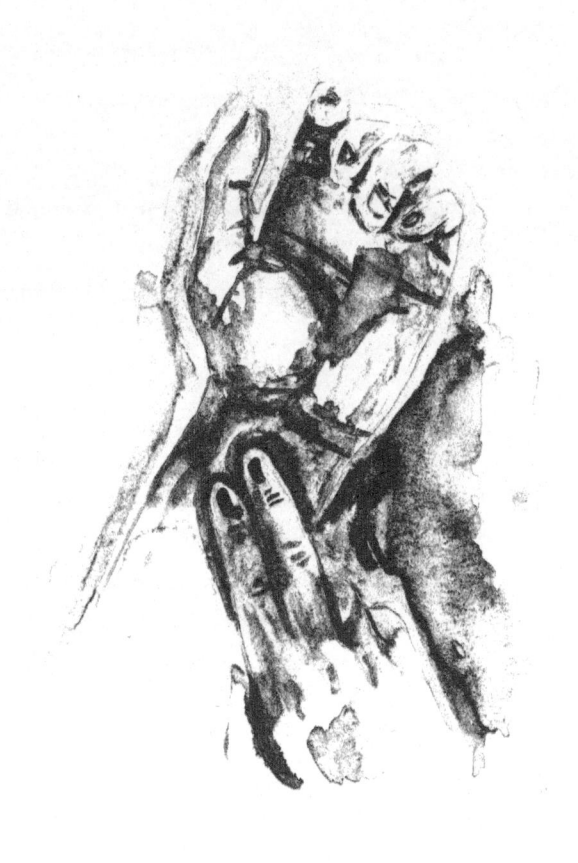

Preface

This book makes significant demands on the reader, but I assume that the reader will be eager to rise to the challenge of backchecking significant names and allusions. *Scattered Limbs* is certainly a text that is meant to be "tasted" in Bacon's phrase, rather than "swallowed"—a book to be opened at random, dipped into, browsed through. Neither index nor footnotes have been provided, since I wanted to avoid what James Joyce called "the true scholastic stink" (without leaving myself in bad odour): most people have access to an encyclopaedia these days at the mere swipe of a phone. Such are the benefits of the codex, whether paper or electronic. One of the major themes of *Scattered Limbs* is the experience of reading itself—reading not just books but bodies, inscriptions and signs. There is nothing deeper than the skin, as Paul Valéry insisted.

Scattered Limbs is a commonplace book, halfway between *zibaldone* and intellectual diary—a miscellany that explores the intermittencies of my relations with the medical profession. It is intended for general readers intrigued by the cultural aspects of medicine, for those puzzled by what political scientists call "the British malaise", for voyeurs at the autopsy table, for those who suspect that the body has become "a shiny artefact of the past" (Leonard Cohen), for the merely curious and even, I dare say, for disillusioned medical practitioners who wonder why medicine, while up for so much in the technological domain, is so thin in self-understanding. Dissatisfaction with medicine is an integral part of the larger discussion about civilisation and its discontents: the conviction of the nineteenth century that all the ills of humankind could be remedied by technical means is still a prevalent one. In its long history medicine has never been spared critics—not when it was ineffective, and not when it became effective, comprehensive and far safer than in the past. In recent years, however, patients have served what they see as an increasingly technocratic profession with a writ of habeas corpus, even as a recent movement has developed among concerned doctors, patients and policy-makers called "Too Much Medicine"—which insists that overdiagnosis and unnecessary care pose a threat to human health (as well as wasting valuable resources).

As a secular stand-in for salvation, medicine now faces a crisis of representation much like that which faced the Church five hundred years ago when Luther's edicts caused Christendom to splinter into competing factions. Something analogous is happening when so many patients opt to receive their "sacraments" from the many practitioners of complementary and alternative medicines while the "true Church" of conventional medicine ever more defensively guards its orthodoxy ("evidence-based medicine"). This is doubly curious since doctors have been steadily relinquishing their traditional roles—away from hierarchies and towards networks—ever since medicine first began to be effective, circa 1850. Treatments work even when patients (and doctors) are blind to their effects. Authority has shifted to the process, away from prestigious persons. "Do we still need doctors?" is a question that would not have arisen, paradoxically, in the era in which doctors were least effective (nearly all of recorded history), but it served as title for an American book published at the turn of the millennium.

I make no claim to be a philosopher except in the etymological sense of the word, but I have tried to catch the pulse of my own time in (scenic) thought, to purloin a well-known phrase by Hegel. *Scattered Limbs* is a book that sticks its neck out, and will not please everyone. But as Henry James said: "I don't want everyone to like me; I should think less of myself if some people did." The future might be gleaming with all kinds of miniaturised gizmos and dematerialised marvels—AI, telemedicine, robot-assisted surgery, genomics, biometry, theranostics and as yet unthought-of interfaces between bodies and machines—but backwards is surely the direction to be facing if we wish to give a true account of how medicine arrived where it has, and indeed of its considerable accomplishments.

The historian Roy Porter once remarked that "we lack proper studies of the cultural meanings of medicine—the place of the doctor, and the resonances of the healing arts, in society." This book might not be altogether "proper" in the historian's sense, but it covers considerable ground, from the startling successes of ancient magical medicine—with several glimpses of the figure of Jesus as healer—to the rarefied atmosphere of Thomas Mann's *Der Zauberberg* in which a fictional character attempts to stay spiritually alive in spite of the surrounding cynicism (and disease), as well as to the political and social ideals behind the British National Health Service that, bucking the trend of the times, allowed general (rather than specialised) medicine to develop and even flourish in corporatist-collectivist Britain in the thirty years after the Second World War.

And while my book—the product of twenty years of observations, comments and arguments, some recruited to counter my own sense of demoralisation—takes issue with the self-images of the profession no less than the streamlined truisms of the age of health, happiness and well-being, I hope its sympathy for the person Virginia Woolf described as "a blown leaf on the edge of time" is still manifest. Composure is a quality that most doctors strive to acquire, although it isn't always easy to maintain. Chekhov once wrote to his patron and publisher Suvorin to explain why: "You need equanimity in this world: only people with equanimity can see things clearly, be fair and work."

The other kind of health

"Health is a state of complete physical, mental and social well-being and not merely the absence of disease or infirmity." So runs the preamble to the Constitution of the World Health Organization as adopted at an international conference in New York in 1946, signed by the representatives of 61 States, and which entered into force (as the bureaucratic expression has it) on 7 April 1948.

The last of the great Bakhtishu family of physicians, around the year 1000 in Baghdad, would have been mystified by this definition (which is regularly cited in the medical literature) since it offers nothing recognisable to a physician. In his treatise *The Medical Garden*, he writes about complexion, psychological states and what is necessary for bodily function.

Then, he writes, there is the other kind of health—an absolute and perfect state, which is the peak of perfection. "This kind does not exist."

Ways to strength and beauty

One of the remarkable crazes around the turn of the twentieth century was the physical fitness movement. It has distinct roots in the politics of Bismarck's Prussia and contributed to the idea that the state ought to invest in the health of its citizens in order for them to be more productive and, in time of ultimate need, able to transform themselves into Spartan soldiers: there was a distinct feeling in France after 1870 that it had lost the war with the upstart nation in the east because it was physically decadent.

Yet the Germans themselves were increasingly prone to feelings of being "lebensmüde" ("tired of life"). Bismarck himself submitted in the early 1880s to a customised diet and physiotherapy at the hands of the physician Ernst Schweninger which successfully transformed him from "an obese and miserable dotard" to new vigour; Schweninger's reward was a professorial chair at the Charité. Friedrich Nietzsche's obsession with his diet was utterly characteristic of the times, as were his complaints about his compatriots' lack of distinction. Degeneration theory developed out of Darwinism and found a promoter in Max Nordau, whose book *Entartung* (*Degeneration*, 1892) had a great effect, not least on twentieth-century political movements. It raised the possibility that terminal exhaustion and decline were conditions being brought on by modernity itself.

Physical fitness was one of the strategies developed to counter this horror of weediness. Millions of men and women across Europe took up callisthenics, gymnastics and other kinds of physical exercise regimes, Franz Kafka for one: every morning with missionary zeal he completed a set of exercises devised by the Danish gym instructor Jørgen Peter Müller in front of an open window and without any special equipment ("Müllerising"). Those who promoted fitness made big claims for it: it would do nothing less than save the world from "physical degeneracy." Müller called his book of exercises "My System", and claimed that he was "physically the most perfect man." Eugen Sandow, Joseph Pilates, Pehr Henrik Ling—these are the names of some of the other pioneers who devised courses of "corrective exercises" to restore a jaded Europe to a physical (and implicitly moral) perfection. Sandow was a circus and music hall performer who invented what we now call "body-building." Pilates, who greatly admired the Greeks, advocated "contrology" and his method, initially taken up by a generation of dancers, is still practised by 11 million people worldwide (including my wife). Yoga made its appearance in the British Empire, and was no longer just a curiosity practised by strange Hindu yogis. There was even a movement called "muscular Christianity," which sought to convert the working classes from seemingly inevitable decline to the healthy sheen of a sweat both physical and spiritual.

Just as neurasthenia made its appearance as a fashionable diagnosis, Sandow's magazine *Physical Culture* promoted the survival of the fittest as a kind of physical prowess and effulgent virility that could be adopted by the individual with regular exercise—body culture as a ritual. This was back to Nature with a vengeance. "Du mußt dein Leben ändern" ("you must change your life") was how the poet Rainer Maria Rilke closed one of his classically themed sonnets. The instruction was out of the bag. The German Lebensreform (Life Reform) movement, Bircher muesli, nudism, vegetarianism, natural medicine and other kinds of political hygiene, free dance and modern dance are all contemporaneous with this wish to return to the apparent simplicities of the body after a century of frenetic industrial production.

The cult of the body manifested itself only when it had ceased to be universally human and had almost imperceptibly given way to a structure that in undertaking minutely defined repetitive tasks produced precisely quantifiable yields, both in factories and in gyms: in other words, a machine. Ergonomics and sports methods don't simply observe the body at work; they provide the very possibility of a notion such as the "body beautiful". It looks aesthetic; it smells of engine oil.

Taking them seriously

Like the militant group Keepers of the Eternal and Victorious Islamic Nation (KEVIN for short) in Zadie Smith's first novel *White Teeth*, WONCA (World Organization of National Colleges, Academies and Academic Associations of General Practitioners/Family Physicians)—whose European congress I once attended in Santiago de Compostela (but not on foot) —has "an acronym problem."

I'm sure the board of WONCA doesn't see it that way: these days an acronym is a guarantee of full corporate existence.

A version of pastoral

Pastoralism is a branch of agriculture and animal husbandry specifically concerned with the care, tending and use of cattle. So what does it have to do with medicine? It is also a form of domestication and social organisation that was incorporated into the text of Christian theology as a model: the good pastor tends his sheep as in Ezekiel 34, and brings his scattered charges together "out from the peoples" and feeds them "in all the habitable places of the country." And the famous parable in Luke 15 even envisages the good shepherd leaving the ninety-nine secure members of his flock in the wilderness and going after the lost sheep until it is found. (Parables are little shrines in the landscape of literature, much visited by pastoralists who know that the concern for the lost sheep isn't driven by statistics.)

Historically, mobile pastoralists have often been at odds with sedentary peoples, and the literature of Bible times is full of their conflicts. Much writing about general practice before the advent of the market in the UK is unselfconsciously written in the pastoral mode, and thereafter in the knowledge that something precious had been lost by adopting the new script for the organisation of society in managerial terms. Friedrich Schiller (who trained as a doctor) defined this kind of nostalgia as "an image of our infancy irrevocably past." Those who write about it, like me, are pastoral theorists. *Et in arcadia ego.*

Perhaps when we get down to it all that is left of pastoralism—if we go back to the source of the great religions with their toppling over-heavy metaphysical superstructures—is a scribbled receipt for sheep. And not necessarily one scribbled by the shepherd either.

"In pastoral," wrote William Empson, preaching on behalf of topical realism in his critical masterpiece *Some Versions of Pastoral*, "you take a limited life and pretend that it is the full and normal one."

Yet some believe it is the condition to which all literature aspires: "Literature will and must always be in the pastoral mode," writes Charles Lock, "in order to be identified as literature."

Unacknowledged

There are stories at the heart of which lie secrets that can never be recounted and words that have the capacity to destroy as well as heal. Parsifal was the knight who, afraid of breaking the rules of courteous engagement and being seen to be fawn or flatter (something no genuine knight would ever do), omitted to ask the troubling question, the word that cuts to the quick, and thereby failed to heal the ailing Fisher King.

One better than Houdini

There's a lovely passage in a volume of Frederic Raphael's diaries which likens his being present at the birth of his daughter to witnessing the ultimate conjuring trick. The room contains n people, notably an expectant mother in some discomfort; nobody comes in, but suddenly there is $n+1$ in the room. I wanted to tell Frederic, with whom I've exchanged the occasional letter, that this is the modern way of expressing what the psalmist says in Psalm 139 about the golem contemplating the God who fashioned his members during many days "when as yet there was none of them."

Angels and prostitutes

A fifteenth-century illuminated manuscript in the Bibliothèque Nationale, Paris, offers an allegory of Mercy offering her breast to a needy patient caught short on the involuntary pilgrimage through life. Providing milk—mother's milk, that precious biofluid—is the primal gift. The Church was not slow to realise that the figure of the Madonna lactans was an immediately intelligible expression of what loving your neighbour actually means.

Ivan Illich comments in his testamental book *The Rivers North of the Future* that the term education, derived from the Latin verb *educare*, is conventionally defined as meaning "to lead out". In fact, in the classical Latin dictionaries, the verb is linked to the suckling of infants: when Cicero writes "nutrix educat", he means that the wet-nurse educates through her milk. This, Illich adds, is what bishops in the early Christian church sought to do for their flock.

The many depictions of the Mercy lending succour in the early modern period (and the Madonna giving breast) express the ambiguity of nursing as a profession: nothing more sublime than such intimately physical succour, nothing more abject than lending your dugs to a stranger.

A LISP

The best thing anybody can say about me is that I am a doctor who has lost his complacency. Unfortunately, I am also a doctor who has lost his patients.

A VISCERAL ATTACHMENT

The female version of the needy and destitute on our streets is called the "bag-lady": her personal effects are usually englobed in five or six plastic bags, some of which may be transported in a caddy. Women as opposed to men have an eye for bags, not least as fashion articles. As rounded receptacles they do seem to be related to aspects of the female anatomy: laps, wombs and breasts.

Perhaps women's bags are actually shields. Or even remonstrations against having to carry so many things, especially children.

When he felt the need to blaspheme the Virgin Mary, Alberto Caeiro—the "shepherd" invented by the Portuguese poet Fernando Pessoa—wrote: "She wasn't even a woman: she was [a] handbag." It took a figure as single-minded as Margaret Thatcher to turn the said appendage into a rhetorical weapon. "To handbag", according to the OED, is "to verbally attack or crush a person or idea ruthlessly and forcefully."

The Serpent and the Staff

It was the Lord Himself who told his people, rather surprisingly in view of the absolute prohibition on image-worshipping and idolatry which characterises the early books of the Bible, to make "a fiery serpent, and set it upon a pole: and it shall pass, that every one that is bitten, when he looketh upon it, shall live" (Numbers 21:8). This was the remedy for the fiery serpents which the Lord had not long before loosed among His people as a punishment for not doing what they had been told to do in the first place. Eventually the people forgot the connection, and the prophet Hezekiah had to have the serpent destroyed—the children of Israel were worshipping it under the name "Nehushtan".

Is this substantially different from the attributes of the serpent and the staff that have come down to us from the cult of Asclepius, the god of healing worshipped by Hippocrates? In a straightforward manner the snake may symbolise renewal and rejuvenation through moulting, in which the growing snake sheds its old skin by rubbing itself against a solid object, causing the cuticle to crack and split open. Some might even see that as a kind of resurrection. Cornutus in his *Theologiae Graecae Compendium* suggested that people who avail themselves of Asclepius' expertise will slough off old age in a manner analogous to the snake. But we know enough, both culturally and biologically, about dealings between humans and the order *Squamata* to suspect that a more ambiguous symbolism is at work. Snakes may symbolise medicine's dealings with both life and death, health and sickness, as well as the ancient understanding of the double-sidedness of the *pharmakon*—the medicine which can kill as well as heal. Snakes also symbolise (in a more occult manner) the baleful hypodermic strike of the sacred, which the market is continually at work attempting to defang.

And there is of course the other symbol, the staff, the walking stick of those doctors who walked the roads and byways of ancient Greece in search of those who needed their help. The staff could fend off the aforementioned snake, should a live one ever be met on the way, since the snake itself is a kind of stick: the stick that moves. (Unless it's frozen: Idris Parry tells the possibly apocryphal story from the Balkans of the peasant struggling home in a snowstorm with a stick found on his path only to discover it stirring when he got back to the safety of his fire.)

Once the itinerant physician had made it to the marketplace in the next town he would be safe. There he fell under the protection of Hermes, the trickster god who smiles on quacks, charlatans, pharmacopolae (retailers of nostrums), street entertainers, mendicant priests and other classes of people with the gift of the gab. Even—according to Lucian of Samosata—those doing a roaring trade in snake-juice.

[Intriguingly, the exceedingly popular, pot-bellied, elephant-headed Hindu god Ganesha, who looks nothing at all like Hermes, is also the god of thieves as well as the patron of the medical profession. You can hardly visit India and not notice Ganesh advertising services on billboards, in plastercast effigy at the next roundabout, twirling his trunk on laminated business cards... He is well-disposed towards humans, and renowned for removing obstacles: this also makes him popular in India with pregnant women.]

Making prognoses

What kind of order would we have if works of fiction were judged in terms of their *prognostic* value?

We may already have moved in this direction, given Kafka's very high contemporary standing. But so many novels which set out expressly to be prescient—Huxley is the best example—come to seem very dated and old-fashioned.

What would prognostic correctness mean? Even when readers recognise certain signs or patterns as leaning into the future, trying to tell us how we will be living then (who is this *we*?), the literary value of a work does not automatically increase. Prognostic abilities rest on the writer's recognition of the universal phenomena expressed by the regularities of social intercourse: the prognosticator has to be an applied sociologist of our second nature. Which means having a theory of origins. As Stanislaw Lem, a writer genuinely learned in axiology, says, "we cannot afford to be spared from reality, no matter how cruel, if we are to remain in the categories of the real world."

Prognostication is where writers and doctors resemble each other most.

Anecdotes

Like literature, medicine started out as an oral history and became so comprehensively a written one that it is easy to forget where it originated. In fact, it teems with a myriad of oral histories—anecdotes. For most of their university training medical students are so immersed in the great master narratives of disease recognition and the burning issues of public health that it almost seems comic to be faced with a patient at all. Indeed, it is only relatively recently in the history of medical teaching that students have been taken systematically to patients' bedsides to learn about the natural history of disease, and even now teaching in some continental European countries still evinces an Olympian disdain for the ungainly mess of the body—empirical and semiological findings are important, but only if they can be abstracted, and doctored up a bit. The overriding problem with patients is that they like to talk, some like to talk a lot, and some even like to talk back.

In their written form, anecdotes (literally "items that have not been published" or "secret histories") are on the whole not taken very seriously by literary critics, even though one of the greatest works of English literature, John Aubrey's *Brief Lives* is appreciatively full of them. Aubrey, who started out as an antiquary, saving objects from the work of time, was criticised by his contemporaries for being "too minute", but he himself was convinced that he was getting at "the naked and plaine trueth", and that the telling detail could yield the essence of a subject. Most of Aubrey's anecdotes are free-standing, flawed and jagged but twitchily alive, full of marginal reminders to himself to check facts and lapses of memory; had he been able to tidy up and polish his prose his book probably wouldn't be read by anyone today except scholars. (I differ here from the French writer Marcel Schwob, who thought Aubrey would have been a greater biographer if he had taken the trouble to establish connections "between individual facts and general actions.")

Anecdotes go in all directions. The sixth-century historian Procopius used anecdotes to hint at the true story of the steamy goings-on at the court of the emperor Justinian—his anecdotes are coded revelations that debunk the glorious official history. Friedrich Schlegel thought that the anecdote was the very ground of the novelistic—"all else is a later transformation." Every one of Heinrich von Kleist's discomfiting stories, with their philosophical and socio-political implications hanging like cobwebs over a measured, implicating, legalistic syntax, derives from anecdotal sources. Heidegger said, with some justification, that anecdotes were the enemy of reason. But just look at Stendhal: his journeys through France and Italy are full of ad libs, as he struggled to reveal—and not only to himself—the mishaps that befall his characters because of a flaw in their understanding of themselves. (And his autobiography *La Vie de Henry Brulard* also profits from being written as a work in progress, its digressions and improvisations and chronological leaps left unrevised.) Nothing quite as effectively points up the difference between the ideal and the real as the well-chosen anecdote. The German philosopher Hans Blumenberg was even prepared to concede that the anecdote can be a genre of philosophical explaining in which "no detail is capricious."

There is a trickster quality to signs or stories that stand at the intersection of two ways of understanding the world, or between public chronicles and private passions. They are written as fragments—brief, closed, hermetic, both a "hole" and a "whole". Anecdotes can be highly conventional, upholders of the world-order just the way it is (moralising media stories and factoids) *and* deeply subversive—accounts of odd events for which the established view of history and perhaps even human nature have no response. These anecdotes find no echo in the vast archives of knowledge. And while they might be secret histories, they never add up to a comprehensive "secret history": anecdotes are contingent reminders that we can't ever fully understand the hidden workings of anything, from the market to God.

In their most subtle form, anecdotes reveal both the forgotten connections that need to be re-established in order to make sense of the past, and the variety, excluding all unity, of that past. Much of modernist art tries to reinvent the anecdote: as Mallarmé put it, "everything happens, truncated, hypothetically; narrative is avoided." The great Russian theorist Viktor Shklovsky even hoped that anecdote—"a story consisting of separate facts tenuously connected"—might replace plot in the conventional novel and allow ideas and events to jostle each other in an aesthetics of disjunction and collision.

Head of Zeus

The latest advances in assisted reproductive technology, with techniques such as gamete donation, pre-implantation genetic diagnosis and cryopreservation, have made it possible for single persons, same-sex couples and even dead persons to reproduce; they suggest that in the future human relations are going to offer a renaissance for the remarkable body morphing that was characteristic of the old polytheistic gods.

Take the story of Zeus and Metis, one of the primordial goddesses in the Greek pantheon. Metis was the daughter of Oceanus and Thetys, the first couple in the Greek pantheon. Metis was cousin to Zeus and his first wife. Hesiod's *Theogony* tells us that Metis helped Zeus to become top god but also presented a threat to his rule: it had been prophesied that she would bear children who would overthrow him. All too keenly aware that he himself had acquired sovereignty by toppling his own father Kronos, Zeus turned Metis into a fly and swallowed her.

What Zeus didn't know was that Metis was already pregnant. As the pregnancy grew it started to cause Zeus considerable discomfort—Metis was somehow lodged in his head (male births have always been head births). Zeus called on the services of the blacksmith god Hephaestus, whose response was to cleave his head with a hammer. The child that emerged was wearing a rather special kind of caul: a full metal helmet.

Zeus was no worse for this drastic self-birthing experience, and his daughter would become famous as Athena, goddess of wisdom and patron of the city of Athens.

And if the future is really going to be full of such chimerical beings, then perhaps we'll need to think more often of Metis. Originally associated with wisdom and deep thought, the Stoic philosophers made *metis* the quality of prudence or good counsel. It was also the epithet most often associated with Odysseus, whose wily intelligence and alert shrewdness led him back home in Homer's other book.

Chekhov's confidence

Anton Chekhov helped to prevent a Russian journal of surgery, *The Surgical Chronicle*, from going under in 1895, fought "the Indian commas" (*vibrio cholerae*, the bacteria which caused cholera), cleaned up the hovels in Talesh, Novosyolki and Melikhova, and ensured the provision of clean water on his estate, under the impress of the conviction that while nature is not benevolent, one could take comfort, much as Thomas Hardy did, in all candour, from human agency and creatureliness—"loving-kindness, operating through scientific knowledge." Both had a subdued good nature which, because their understanding of the world was sober, not to say grim, shines through the gloom.

Small deaths

Tiraqueau, an acquaintance of the great François Rabelais, had it in his Laws of Marriage, that Hippocrates ("the greatest of doctors") considered "that sexual coitus is part of that terrifying illness which the Greeks calls *epilepsia* and the Latins *morbus comitialis.*" Presumably he was thinking of its paroxysmal phase: Galenic medicine believed that sperm originated in the brain. Moralists were able to dine out on this idea for two millennia, and the conceit had a related existence in the idea of orgasm as a small death.

In his great poem *The Exstasie* John Donne defines the sexual climax as "unperplexing": it undoes us, and we undo ourselves—in the recurrent act that "diminisheth the length of life a day".

In most European languages, men and women "come" at the paroxysmal moment. Shakespeare made his Egyptian Queen declare that she is dying to come: in the last act of *Antony and Cleopatra*, Cleopatra tells her maids in sexually heightened language of her desire for union with her dead husband: "Husband, I come." She is sure to arrive at the predestined place.

Contrast that with Hungarian and Malay (and perhaps in other languages beyond my ken) where sexual partners "leave" when they climax, a notion even more suggestive of self-dissolution.

And the moral-physiological idea that orgasm literally shortens life, that to ejaculate is to squander the life-force—a version of the notion that the more you take from life the less remains to be lived—in a persistent belief among writers: Hemingway firmly believed he only had "so many shots in the bucket." Balzac adhered to a kind of finite vitalism too: sperm was an emission of the purest thought. He once turned up at a friend's house, having spent the evening with a voluptuous creature, exclaiming: "I just lost a book!" This is the hydraulic vision of desire found in Freud's writing, too: libidinal capital is stocked in a kind of reservoir, and if you open the sluice gates of sexuality then the spirit level of the sublime suffers.

Other cultures have plenty of superstitions about the nature of semen: in India it is widely believed that one drop of the stuff is equivalent to forty drops of blood. Taoism and Tantric yoga impose strictures on its adherents on the grounds of this belief as well: Sanskrit texts suggest that semen must not be emitted if the yogi seeks to avoid falling under the law of time and death.

Books have been written on the ingenious physical methods that were formerly employed to prevent onanism. The Victorian age was particularly obsessed with the figure of the lantern-jawed, slack-eyed, pallid-skinned teenage masturbator, the young man who had dared to play fast and loose with Lord Thomson's Second Law of Thermodynamics and phallus in hand was gratuitously dissipating all the energy and industry of the universe.

There are of course a few admirable spendthrifts who live in the conviction that the more you take from life the less will be left for death.

A GENUFLECTION

Not the heart but the knees: the religious "organ" develops pads. These bits of our anatomy are known in medicine as the infrapatellar fat pads of Hoffa.

Ludwig Wittgenstein's knees, he confessed in a letter, were too "stiff" for him to develop prayer pads. He wasn't going to adopt Pascal's "we must kneel, pray with the lips, &c.", so that the bend of his knee would make plain the genuflection of his soul ("Inclina cor meum. Deus!"). Wittgenstein wanted a God who would see, without the need for external evidence, that he had submitted his spirit to the letter.

W. H. Auden said prayer was listening, and that it could become a serious habit only once the petitioner had stopped making begging requests. Praying persons listened for the Voice, which "always says something new and unpredictable—an unexpected demand, obedience to which involves a change of self, however painful".

Charles Baudelaire also believed in the efficacy of prayer. That is why he resolved, every morning, to pray to the souls of his father, his governess and Edgar Allan Poe.

The world is round

Without apoptosis (Greek: "dropping off") or programmed cell death, a phenomenon which was first described in 1842, we would not be able to develop fingers and limbs. More than 50 billion cells die each day in the adult human organism on account of this phenomenon, and although that might sound an overwhelming quantity it represents a mere fraction of the total body cell population. Cell death is of course offset by proliferation. Over a year, however, the number of cells shed amounts to approximately our total body weight: without apoptosis we would be true blubber monsters with 16 kilometres of intestines and bones weighing hundred-weights—something like the spherical ideal beings in Plato's *Timaeus* but not nearly so perfectly hermetic and morphologically desirable.

Leonardo da Vinci's famous citation, "Our life is made by the death of others", could therefore be modified to read: "Our life is made by the death of our own substance."

A major incompatibility syndrome

Being an intellectual dandy and a general practitioner is about as likely a combination as being an intellectual dandy and a family man. It is also known as the Oscar Wilde syndrome.

Marxists and the market

The last few years have seen the appearance of several books criticising what has been called therapy culture, barely noticed against the hundreds of books insisting, on the other hand, that being ill can be a unique learning opportunity.

What's intriguing about this critical trend—certainly more of an intellectual than a popular movement—is that many of its leading theorists are former Marxists, chief among them Frank Furedi, professor of sociology at the University of Kent and former chairman of the Revolutionary Communist Party. These critics observe that therapy culture has replaced religion as the opium of the people, illness has become a first-order experience and health comprehensively politicised; and that consequently we have entered a kind of arms race of public emoting.

None of these are false observations; yet the suspicion remains that critics of such stripe are motivated by ideological reasons and less by an old-fashioned desire to recover the fortitude that marked an earlier generation. Their philosophy of unlimited progress seems as misplaced and unrealistic as that of those who aspire to victim status. If only the people weren't so narcotised by being "healthy" and actually got around to overthrowing the state...

LI MEDICI ME CREARONO E DISTRUSSONO

In a pun scribbled in his notebook concerning his patron Lorenzo Medici and the medical profession ("I medici"), Leonardo da Vinci became one of the first thinkers to advance the understanding— later associated with Goethe's *Faust* and thereafter with the economist Schumpeter—that creativity and destruction are intimate allies. In Leonardo's eyes physicians practised a killing and not a healing art since they preyed on those with infirmities and ailments.

THE BODY OF POWER

Most of the comments on the film adaptation of Giles Foden's novel *The Last King of Scotland* see it as a straightforward moral tale about what happens when a politically naive but energetic young Scottish doctor, Nicholas Garrigan, doing medical relief work in a bush hospital in Uganda, encounters the head of state, Idi Amin, in person—that is His Excellency President for Life Field Marshall Al Hadj Doctor Idi Amin Dada, VC, DSO, MC, Lord of All the Beasts of the Earth and Fishes of the Sea and Conqueror of the British Empire in Africa in General and Uganda in Particular.

Impressed by the young doctor's practical approach to immediate trauma care, and long an admirer of Scottish (military) traditions, Amin invites him to become his personal physician in Kampala. At first things go swimmingly well, but little by little even the self-absorbed Garrigan (the novel is based on a real-life soldier who became Amin's closest adviser) has to face up to the fact that the hypochondriac whose petty illnesses he gets up to treat in the night is also a tyrant with a penchant for the most ridiculous and outrageously brutal whims. This doctor gets off on the thrill of danger: he even has an adulterous affair with the dictator's third and youngest wife, a tryst which gets her butchered and almost costs him his own life.

It would be wrong to assume that it is pure naivety which brings Garrigan to discover his own heart of darkness. Historically, physicians reached the apex of power by ministering to the body of power itself. This becomes clear in the film when Garrigan expeditiously relieves Amin of abdominal cramps during a severe bout of flatulence and for the first time senses the physical danger he has placed himself in: he has ridiculed—albeit inadvertently—the royal body. Those who heal princes and potentates are bound to be raised into relationships of power themselves, just as they can be cast down with them. But it is still not enough to make him aware of his own moral temporising. "I heard him calling himself the last rightful king of Scotland again on the radio," writes Garrigan in the novel, "I thought, in a wild moment, that it had some special relevance for me. As if I were his subject." Which, of course, he is. Amin is astute enough to make the fey Garrigan his factotum, and assign him the ministerial task (for which he has absolutely no qualifications) of overseeing the architectural designs of a conference hall for the next Pan-African Congress.

Things go horribly wrong in Uganda, and Garrigan is lucky to escape with his life. But he is so smugly self-absorbed that the film ends on an uncomfortable note: can a doctor tend such atrocious hurts and wounds without suffering a ricochet injury himself?

Foden's first novel is a variant on a type familiar during the high imperial era: one in which a young man both proves and improves himself by "going out" to Africa or India. His fictional hero has a little in common with John Buchan's David Crawfurd who, in *Prester John*, set in the immediate aftermath of the Anglo-Boer War, engages on a process of discovery, learning and maturation, eventually escaping at improbable odds from a situation that threatens the Empire itself. Initially considered a boys' adventure story *Prester John* has since grown up, now being considered in the same breath as Buchan's other novels. Post-colonialism still offers lots of scope for self-absorbed young innocents in search of adventure: they merely have to flag their humanitarian credentials and one day, if they're lucky, they might just end up being Foreign Minister—of their own improbable and irrelevant kingdom.

A GLIB PHILOSOPHY

The philosopher Epicurus missed the point when he demoted the fear of death to a chiasmatic trick of the tongue: "When I am, death is not, and when death is, I am not"— thereby "exchanging one vacuity for another," as a more modern philosopher jibed. The most difficult thing we must face in life isn't our own death but that of those we love.

TAKE UP YOUR BED

Which Spanish hospital these days would dare to call itself Hospital de la Resurrección, like the institute for syphilitics outside the city gates of Valladolid at which the dogs Scipio and Berganza have their dialogue in Cervantes' famous story? Or French hospital still grandstand as Hôtel-Dieu? Even then there must have been a certain ironic discrepancy between the soaring titles, and the wreckage of human life cast within their walls. People lost things in such places, sometimes their limbs, very often their lives. Hospitals were there to usher you into eternity.

Yet as that great scholar and notable hypochondriac Guido Ceronetti writes, at such places (he has in mind the Pellegrinaio of Santa Maria della Scala in Siena) where the sick congregated there was a caravan of life, a bustle of noisy, swarming, vivid intercourse. Now, he notices, such places with their enormous windows have become sterile whitewashed sepulchres. They have lost any kind of transcendent appeal and are merely refrigerators.

The paradox remains a keen one: that our modern hospital centres owe their existence to a way of thinking that set a higher value on pity (*misericordia*) and charity (*caritas*) than the mere art of healing.

Crafts

Neither the ancient Greeks nor their gods—who were quite often hopelessly wayward in their godliness, not to say downright double-crossing and bed-swapping, and not in the least trustworthy in that long-running soap opera on Mount Olympus—allowed themselves any idea of perfectibility other than the kind of technical perfection that can be developed in a lifetime's application and devotion to a manual skill or *techne*, among which Plato includes medicine, horsemanship, huntsmanship, herding, farming, calculation, geometry, generalship, piloting a ship, chariot-driving, political craft, prophecy, music, lyre-playing, flute-playing, painting, sculpture, housebuilding, shipbuilding, carpentry, weaving, pottery, smithing and cookery.

Seeking to be self-sufficient in the modern manner of Jean-Jacques Rousseau, or to be perfectly happy in the manner of almost everyone after him, was to vaunt "spiritual pride" or hubris—and hubris, like honey to flies, calls down the unfavourable attention of the gods. But throughout the Industrial Revolution, the crafts enjoyed a renaissance as a reaction to the crushing anonymity of the industrial process. "Craft" was the call of rebellion for polemicists from Ruskin and Morris to Loos and Gropius.

It was only after the industrial-scale slaughter of the First World War, when the machine seemed to have won, that the word "craft" became derisory—a pastime for eccentrics and the slightly loopy.

Panicology

Panic is older than the sense of apocalypse that entered Christendom through the dire visions of John of Patmos and the Jewish prophets, far older than the calculating self-interest of *homo economicus*. Our lives no longer reach out to the ultimate consummation of their meaning in the revelation at the end of history, the expectation of which fuelled two thousand years of European civilisation, and lapse instead into terror and blind flight—or what the German novelist Hermann Broch called a "negative ecstasy." We are infected by signs of alarm in others, and we react as they do: there is so little understanding in what we do that we imagine the act originates with us. Panic is the fear of death—not the fear of a natural death but one at the hands of the members of our own culture. Consequently, as the nature of what we now call mass society became more distinct in the twentieth century, as its mediation became more rapid through radio and television, there was a corresponding awakening of interest in the old Greek god: Peter Pan is his most frivolous, flightiest manifestation.

Among his other attributes, the Greek god Pan, with his goatish hindquarters and wild rustic sallies on the flute, was the god of shepherds. He was also the god of wooded groves, glens and the pastures of Arcadia, that unspoiled wilderness in the centre of the Peloponnese. But Pan had other, less commendable traits. He was an insatiable lecher who terrified the nymphs. And he was also the god of midday, when the light at the centre of the natural world itself acts on the unprotected human figure like a blast of revelation so intense as to make it shiver uncontrollably.

Panic (*panikon deima*) is contagious. And for it to strike, humans have to be glued together. This creates the conditions for Jean Baudrillard's "viral hospitality"—or what the Bible calls "legion." A common danger creates a common fear. Lack of differentiation is itself the crisis, and one that can be overcome only by obeying imperatives that are themselves critical. The aversion people normally have to being touched is overcome: they even seek out physical contact. Fire (the heat of midday that makes us shiver) is the very symbol of its movement. And yet we shiver all the more uncontrollably because while we feel the pressing need to separate ourselves from the crowd (where the peril has its source) we cannot, because our whole modern socialisation has insisted on our identification with that same society. We know ourselves to be vulnerable; the panic grows instantly; we trample others (in order to quench the fire); and then we find ourselves bereft.

And as a witty scientist observes in Elizabeth Kolbert's book on the cultural history of extinction, "the history of life consists of long periods of boredom interrupted occasionally by panic." It is the same panic we find in that most ancient of texts, the Veda.

FIXATIVES

The ability to synthesise dyes from coal tar—a development pioneered by German companies like Bayer, Hoechst and BASF after the chemist F. F. Runge managed to product aniline in 1834, an aromatic amine with a benzene ring and amino group—transformed the colours of the average middle-class wardrobe at the end of the nineteenth century, but also provided staining substances that could be used in histology.

Hundreds of stains would be developed including alizarin, alcyan yellow and tartrazine, and they were used to render parts of the cell structure more distinctively vibrant and easier to visualise microscopically—indeed some cell structures were now perceived for the first time. The eosin technique developed by the Russian pathologist Romanowsky was the forerunner of several related methods such as the Giemsa, Jenner and Leishman stains, which were developed to differentiate cells in their medium. Staining techniques indirectly gave rise to the new field of bacteriology (where the preferred stain was methylene blue), and established haematology as a proper specialisation. The famous scientist Paul Ehrlich, who invented the technique that led to Gram staining, was one of the first researchers to study new synthetic dyes systematically and suggest diagnostic uses for them—in the treatment of malaria for instance.

These same dyes were also to give rise to the first real set of new elements in the pharmacopoeia, including acetanilide. It was another dye, Prontosil rubrum (Prontosil red), discovered by a German biochemist Gerhard Domagk in 1935 and produced after modification by the German firm later to become infamous as IG Farben as the "sulfa" antibiotics, that gave medicine its first real "magic bullet" (a notion popularised by Ehrlich). Some dyes—the previously mentioned methylene blue, which because it turns the urine blue was used for decades by physicians as a placebo—also proved to be crucial, after the Second World War, in the development of antipsychotics and antidepressants.

The dispensation

General practice in the United Kingdom between 1950 and 1980 was a realisation of John Ruskin's great dream in *Fors Clavigera* (1871-1884), the series of ninety-six jeremiads and hortatory letters he addressed to British workmen in the 1870s—a vision of a heaven of handicrafts. The "dignity of craft" vision did not appeal to everyone: H. G. Wells, son of a draper, once commented that it needed "the Olympian unworldliness of an irresponsible rich man of the shareholding type, a Ruskin or a Morris, playing at life" to advance such a high-minded notion. Nonetheless, while a very mid-twentieth-century esteem for scientific language and values (the social-scientific background espoused by the early Labour Party and advanced by Wells too) might have ousted the trades-guild medievalism that appealed so much to Ruskin, in other respects doctors and nurses continued to uphold a British sense of social life as *pantomime*—which is to theatrical life what ritual is to church life (as illustrated in those once popular Doctor in the House comedies starring Dirk Bogarde). It may well be that the National Health Service was the last major institution to be forged by what some historians call British society's "patriotic Protestant foundation-myth."

With time, however, something soured as people generally became better off: more and more patients came in speaking

Pinterese, or took their cue from continental dramas—Brecht's agitprop or the Theatre of the Absurd (*The King Departs*). Then pantomime restored itself, though the plot was a different one: the wicked Stepmother known as Mrs Thatcher turned up brusquely in the last act and announced a new nativity.

Yet the new nativity was the old one that had so appalled Ruskin. It was the dance around the Golden Calf.

The trick is to keep breathing

Making elaborate statements of the bleeding obvious: that is the chief skill of Eryximachus, the vain doctor in *The Symposium*. And offering cures for hiccoughs.

A new sophism

David Hume in his introduction to *A Treatise of Human Nature* sounds uncommonly modern. Disputes are multiplied, as if everything was uncertain; and these disputes are managed with skill and assurance, as if everything was certain.

Amid all this bustle, it is not reason which carries the prize, but eloquence; and no man need ever despair of gaining proselytes to the most extravagant hypothesis, if he is skilled enough to represent it in a favourable colour.

Victory is gained not by the men at arms, those who wield the instruments of powers but by the trumpeters, drummers and regimental musicians.

Money (that's what I want)

Profits from The Beatles records in the late 1960s were so substantial that EMI (Electrical and Musical Industries Ltd.) was able over four years to fund Godfrey Hounsfield's attempts to develop a computed tomography (CT) scanner at its research labs in Hayes, Middlesex. The original 1971 prototype took 160 parallel readings each one degree apart, with every scan taking just over 5 minutes. It then took 150 minutes to process the images by algebraic reconstruction on a large scanner. The introduction of *depth* to the radiological image was the single most revolutionary step in radiology since the discovery of X-rays by Roentgen himself in 1896, the CT scanner being the first imaging device to allow detailed visualisation of the internal anatomy of living creatures in three dimensions as distinct from the X-ray which offers solely two-dimensional radiodense shadows. A CT-slice image is composed of voxels (volume elements) by analogy with the pixels (picture elements) of a digital image.

CT scanners were calibrated with reference to distilled water, which at a standard pressure and temperature was assigned a radiodensity of zero Hounsfield units: this allowed a linear scale to be constituted as a universally applicable reference for imaging the internal structure of living creatures (lung − 700 HU, cancellous bone + 700 HU). It was based on the fact that we are to a remarkable extent living structures in which water and air have been organised and partitioned.

SPECIALISTS, EXPERTS AND LEARNED DONKEYS

Jean Paul, in his novel *Doktor Katzenbergers Badereise* or *Dr Katzenberger's Journey to the Spa* (1809), is generally credited with marking the first appearance of a *Fachidiot*, the very type of a narrow-minded or blinkered specialist. "Jeder Fachmann ist in seinem Fach ein Esel"—an expert can become so overspecialised as to be a dolt, even in his profession.

Those days must have seen a plague of such doctors, since many turn up in nineteenth-century literature, most memorably perhaps in Georg Büchner's play *Woyzeck*, and Goya even portrays a donkey-doctor in Capricho 42, titled "You who cannot?"—Watteau has the pairing too, at the bottom of his famous Pierrot: they were standard pantomime figures of commedia dell'arte. What characterises the *Fachidiot* is his stupidity in cleverness, and extreme emotional detachment from the ordinary implications of acting on his special knowledge. He is "double-blinded" in a rather special way.

Later in the nineteenth century Marx took up the French term "*idiotisme du métier*" to describe the effects of the division of labour on modern society, a phenomenon which Ruskin railed against too; but it was surely the benefits provided by compartmentalisation that Nietzsche had in mind when he wrote, tongue in cheek, in *Human, All too Human*, "A profession makes us thoughtless: that is its greatest boon. It is a bulwark, behind which we are allowed to withdraw when qualms and worries of a general kind assail us."

Nietzsche had been an academic philologist long enough to understand what he was talking about. Professions in the modern era are cloistered forms of living that are subject to close surveillance and as jealously guarded as private property.

Too close for comfort

There's a nicely observed moment in Gavin Francis' book *Adventures in Human Being* that captures what happens when a doctor performs fundoscopy with a handheld ophthalmoscope, which requires him, the examiner, to stand jowl to cheek with the patient so that he can illuminate and study the back of the eyeball: both parties hold their breath because they suddenly realise they have overstepped the unacknowledged but inviolable code that keeps us at arm's length in social intercourse: this is too close for comfort in a non-intimate relationship. Civilisation is all about distance and equipoise.

Retinal exams are now done largely by sophisticated cameras, with automated image processing: MIT's Media Lab has developed software to analyse retinal colour, blood-vessel shape and other signs and stigmata. Manual fundscopy, which is a sophisticated examination itself, suddenly appears very old-fashioned—like the general practitioners who are competent to use such devices. I remember that one of my shock moments in

France was attending an educational evening where a specialist ophthalmologist had to explain to the assembled *généralistes* what an ophthalmoscope was, and how it was used.

A LOOPHOLE

I wondered once if the verb in the old Scots expression, "Ah cannae thole it"—which was blurted out by the patient who came to the surgery in Wigtownshire in distress one afternoon and then repeated herself for my benefit in standard English when she remembered I wasn't a local—somehow derived from the Latin phrase "hoc mihi dolet".

I wasn't so foreign as not to have understood her opening phrase, but I didn't let on. She wasn't there for language lessons. "Thole", it turned out once I'd examined her and sent her away with a prescription, doesn't derive from "this pains me": it is cognate with Old Norse "thola" and Middle Low German "dolle", and related to a different Latin verb, "tollere"—although the "dol" root seems to be an Indo-European constant for any painful sensation. A group of doctors at the University of Cornell in the 1940s tried to create a 21-point scale based on the "dol" as a unit of pain experience, blind to the notion of pain as a phenomenon inflected by the tides of culture and context.

"Thole" was one of Seamus Heaney's childhood words— Ulster being just across the water from Galloway—and it seems to have been laden for him with a particular freight of sense, like the Northern Irish exclamation "Och!" which expressed "an Icelandic saga attitude, a fatal sense of how things are". He writes in the introduction to his translation of *Beowulf* that this humble verb was a "little epiphany". It was "the word that older and less educated people would have used in the country where I grew up" (County Derry), and he recalled an aunt saying of a family afflicted by a sudden bereavement, "They'll just have to learn to thole." The stoical tenor is clear enough. What made the word an "illumination by philology" for Heaney was its doubling as a noun: in addition to being associated with suffering and bearing up it denotes the locked upright fitting on the gunwales of a boat in which the oar pivots: the thole-pin.

The oar rubs and rubs at the eyelet which in resisting becomes the fulcrum that allows the boat to shift. As Heaney explains in the introduction to his translation of *Beowulf*, it was this word that gave him the keys to the kingdom.

The Zimmermann Boy

It sounds like a taunt, but Jesus's famous saying was part of a longer phrase addressed to the people of his hometown Nazareth—"Ye will surely say unto me this proverb: Physician, heal thyself." (Luke 4:23). Cyril of Alexandria even calls it a "witticism", and states that it was a common saying among the Jews of the time. The Nazareans wanted to know why this man who was being acclaimed in the region as a spiritual healer, exorcist and preacher could perform miracles and do mighty work in the neighbouring town of Capernaum but not in Nazareth, where he was merely Joe-the-carpenter's boy. ("And brother of James, and Joseph, and Simon, and Judah," and possibly two or three unmentioned sisters.) Until only a short time before, he had been a carpenter himself. And what could a childless man of thirty know about life? (Albrecht Dürer captures this sense of the abashed young Jesus in his painting *Christ among the Doctors*.) The Nazareans thought he had lost his marbles (Mark 3:21).

Jesus was saying they would tell him to save his reputation by proving what he said was true, the implication being that he ought first to cast out his own demons before he could presume to cast out other people's. As Geza Vermes writes, sickness, sin and the devil were interconnected realities for the Jews of antiquity. Not having any demons, Jesus refused to oblige, and reminded them that prophets are never recognised by people who have known them with a snotty nose and schoolbag: "A prophet is not despised except in his own country, and among his own kind, and in his own house." Jesus was unable to do any ministry there apart from healing a few infirm people. After general uproar in the local village hall, the Nazareans decided to throw him off the hilltop on which Nazareth is built, but being a carpenter the King of the Jews must have cut a hole in the floor and made good his escape, passing—as the gospel says—"through their midst."

And this business of stealthily drilling through entrenched positions, as the sociologist Max Weber would agree, is the very nature of politics.

OUR NEWEST COLONY

"My body is that part of the world which my thoughts can alter. Even imaginary illnesses can become real ones. In the rest of the world my hypotheses cannot disturb the order of things." The German philosopher Georg Christoph Lichtenberg was describing, two hundred years ago, the advent of neurasthenia, chronic fatigue syndrome and even mild depression long before such media-transmitted (and possibly even media-generated) syndromes became pervasive in Western culture. We have entered an unparalleled historical situation where the impress of the imagination, multiplied a hundredfold by the products of digital technology, has become so vivid, compelling and ultimately contagious, that reality seems at best a strangely grey and recalcitrant hindrance to its limitless expansion.

And the most unfortunate thing is that these imaginary, metaphorical illnesses produce *real* suffering. They follow the logic of the McGuffin, an empty object, false idea or non-event introduced into a story which nonetheless has real effects. Alfred Hitchcock—who invented the term—knew that these lures left hanging about in the storyline for the purpose of moving it on can sometimes be more compelling than the prosaic truth.

DOMESTIC BLISS

With the demonstration of the bacteria causing typhus, cholera and tuberculosis in the 1880s, and the gradual acceptance of the germ theory of disease thereafter, public health reforms were given a mandate for change.

Germ theory also revolutionised the domestic sphere: thick carpets, drapery and even Victorian wallpaper were no longer compatible with hygiene. Bathrooms and kitchens changed radically. Nonporous materials were developed for flooring and work surfaces, squat legs were slimmed down on stoves and appliances, and heavy furniture disappeared, to be replaced with fixtures. The loose array of moveable chambers pots, washing tubs and washstands was replaced with fixed porcelain-enamelled appliances: dirt could be identified with the naked eye and eliminated. Indoor plumbing became middle-class "American standard" in the 1920s. Thought went into making the kitchen an efficient work space, and the ship's galley design, which had been common in the mid-1800s, was replaced by modular fitted kitchens ready to house the new packaged products of the developing food industry.

Hygiene thus became an integral aspect of the home's "erogenous zones", those settings that do most to create a sense of cleanliness amid grime, intimacy amid otherness, pleasure amid shame. You'll forgive me if I tell you how often I sense a glacier brooding on the other side of bliss.

JOINING THE RIGHT GUILD

To make himself eligible for election to public office in his natal city at the end of the thirteenth century, Dante, as a member of the minor aristocracy, had to join one of Florence's trade guilds. He chose to enrol among the members of the Guild of Physicians and Apothecaries, a trade guild which also happened to incorporate the Papermakers.

The poet cannot claim membership in any guild, says Novalis. Now it is apparent that nobody—in *any* profession—is entirely protected in what we have come to call the global market. The poet knows what it is to exist on the margins; and it is a curious coincidence that now the market obliges us all to live as self-entrepreneurs we have ceased to listen much at all to those voices from before the age of universal literacy.

An uproar

I opened the door and couldn't believe my ears: hundreds of symptoms were all talking back at their diagnostician. A tribe wanted to know if I was their ethnographer.

Men who thought they were Napoleon

Laure Murat in her study of the Paris alienist hospital records shows that, after 1815, acute personality disorder in France manifested itself most commonly as a form of identification with the fallen Emperor. Scores of Napoleons were brought to the asylums every time there was an event connected with his legend, and almost all of them were men—overbearing, short-tempered, severe and authoritarian ("monomanie orgueilleuse"), and often with hand tucked in waistcoat. It was always Bonaparte. Nobody, it seems, ever thought he was the bourgeois emperor, Napoleon III: the mad had a discriminating sense of where true prestige lay.

The reappearances went further than the madhouse. As the writer Philippe Muray insists, "The entire nineteenth century was in a state of delirium around the ghost of Napoleon, to whom a variety of supernatural qualities were attributed." In rural France in particular, sightings of the emperor rivalled those of the Virgin Mary, and there were persistent rumours, as reported by local administrators, of his return at the head of a colossal subterranean army.

Murat considers the possibility that Napoleon might indeed have had a personality disorder himself, and there are certainly plenty of hints that he, like a lot of famous people, had difficulties in disentangling his person from his legend. Balzac comes to mind. And of course, the famous neurologist Jean-Martin Charcot, whose clinical acumen was compared by almost all his *chefs de clinique* at the Pitié-Salpétrière to Bonaparte's strategic genius. (A dubious compliment for a doctor, surely, when we recall that under Napoleon's command, around a million conscripts lost their lives, as many as were killed in the Great War, and a major reason for France's population decline in the nineteenth century relative to the other European powers. Paul Valéry caught the man in a mordant phrase: "He lived off his time – to the point of exhausting it.")

Simon Leys' brief novel *La Mort de Napoléon* (1986) even has the exiled Bonaparte escaping from St Helena with a couple of thousand troops and returning to metropolitan France, only to be incarcerated in an asylum in which all the other denizens are versions of himself. The surrogate who has gallantly taken the place of the fallen emperor on Saint Helena has unfortunately died, perhaps even of natural causes, and now nobody believes this odd man who claims to be the fallen emperor, although he does bear a remarkable likeness to him.

And one of the most famous people to identify with Napoleon wasn't even French. He was in his study at Jena, with the sound of cannon ringing in his ears. His projection was even more extraordinary: it was the sight of this one man he called the "Weltseele" ("world-soul") riding through the city reconnoitring—"a single point [...] reaching out over the world and dominating it". Bonaparte hadn't heard of Professor Hegel and had no plans to visit him.

A BIG BARREL OF HUMANITY

Doctors, male doctors at any rate, seem to be more trustworthy when they are stout. In one of his letters to his fiancée Felice, the tubercular Franz Kafka wrote that he was the leanest person he knew—"I ought to know," he added, "because I've spent a lot of time in sanatoriums and such places"—but went on to remark that he had overcome his habitual distrust of doctors after meeting one who was so stout that "one had to have confidence in him."

W.H. Auden (whose father was a doctor) wrote that he wanted his personal doctor to be "partridge-plump,/ Short in the leg and broad in the rump"—an "endomorph with gentle hands" who would never preach the virtues of being healthy or make a drama out of crisis, and who would tell him straight when he had to pay the ferryman but "with a twinkle in his eye."

A proper attitude to death can be a source of life. That is medicine's only profundity. Provided you can find a doctor who thinks that far ahead. (And one who isn't also in competition with colleagues to usher you over the threshold, like those who attend Mrs Dombey in Dickens' novel. Time may be running out for her, but it is the doctors' timepieces which jump out of fob-pockets and become ensnarled: "The race in the ensuring pause was fierce and furious. The watches seemed to jostle, and to trip each other up.")

What's yours?

Alain de Botton has, I read, made 7 million pounds so far (2014) in his career of bamboozling credulous readers into believing that philosophy is an alternative medicine when it's really a hard drug.

The FT columnist Harry Eyres pointed out in one of his excellent articles in that paper's weekend edition that Krishnamurti is an unsettling philosopher because "he seems to leave you with less than you thought you had, not more." He goes on to observe that this cuts across the capitalist logic that we always get a return on our investment: thinking may not offer any kind of comforts at all, especially if it brings us to wander into some uncharted inhospitable desert in the very next neighbourhood rather than provide the "absolute safety" that loomed so large for Wittgenstein.

In a critical state

Medicine is at heart a philosophical discipline as Galen suggested in his tract, way back in the year 180 (*That the Best Physician is Also a Philosopher*). Contemporary doctors are rarely thinkers, not anymore—time for reflection is swallowed up by the need to act. "Qui ne sait agir n'est pas médecin," wrote Jean Starobinski, the most distinguished member of the Geneva School: he has a doctorate in medicine as well as in letters.

This is the obverse of the situation sarcastically described by the philosopher Søren Kierkegaard: "The secret of life, if you want to get on well in it, is plenty of gossip about what you intend to do and how you're kept from doing it—and no action."

The bottom line would seem to be: if you don't know what to do or how to do it, you're no doctor. The patient might be in a perfect crisis but so too is the doctor: the adjective "critical" alludes to decision-making, a decisive moment—a "cut" as they so rightly say in the cinema.

This is confirmed by the earliest citation of the word in the OED: "Crisis sygnifieth iudgement". It derives from a medical treatise published in 1543.

Lost in action

Paul Valéry likened his working method as a poet-philosopher to that of the surgeon. "In every matter, and before every scrutiny of the core issues, I examine language: it is my habit to proceed like surgeons who disinfect first their hands and prepare the operating field. It is what I call cleansing the verbal situation (*"nettoyage de la situation verbale"*). Forgive me this expression which assimilates the words and forms of discourse to the hands and instruments of an operator" (Zaharoff lecture at Oxford University, 1939).

But the analogy falls flat in one respect. Thought presupposes something at its origin that is more than itself. It is unable to complete itself, and therefore falls short of its actual foundation, existence.

Q&A

"Why me?" demand so many. To which, alas, the only possible answer is: "Why *not* you?"

The realisation that reality is supremely indifferent to our suffering is so unbearable we prefer to think, in an archaic reflex, that external forces are actively hostile and conspiring against us, since this at least puts us in some kind of relation with the world and obliges us to mend the breach. Nobody likes to sleep with the thought that there's nothing for it: we can't be helped. Anthropomorphic convictions give sense and meaning to our lives.

Many people (and not only statisticians) understand the notion of contingency *theoretically*, but few indeed would be prepared to treat their own impending demise with such throwaway disdain as the ailing Paul Valéry. His response was: "Je suis foutu et je m'en fous" ["I'm done for and I don't give a damn", although the French idiom is stronger]. Guido Ceronetti claims even a religious spirit could find his phrase, in its realisation of the ineluctable, "exemplary".

Ceronetti knew Valéry to be a man without religious conviction or solace but found something admirable about the poet's refusal to mourn the loss of (being) nobody but himself.

The drawing board

Those studies of surgeons being gowned up, discussing cases and working on orthopaedic patients—*Concentration of Hands II, Prelude II*—done by Barbara Hepworth in the late 1940s offer some of the most sympathetic portraits of doctors at work. Medical artwork often tends either towards the mawkish (Norman Rockwell) or the brutal (Otto Dix). Many doctors themselves exhibit a bit of both qualities, but Hepworth captures something unique, the total absorption in the task at hand which exemplifies the practical side of medicine.

We ought to be grateful, in an odd way, that marble was in short supply in Britain after the war, since abstract sculpture was where Hepworth thought her talent lay. She had spent the 1920s carving severely distended nudes in a style that owed much to Aristide Malliol, female nudes with very large hands, and then somehow got lost at the end of the following decade in the international religion of geometric abstraction: Carrara marble, as one critic says, "brought out the worst in Hepworth". Her surgical studies, by contrast, offer a series of portraits of socialist medicine at its finest done by an artist who clearly knew her Piero della Francesca (observe the eye of the masked face of the surgeon in *Prevision*, 1948, and the personages who boldly hold our gaze in the Italian master's frescoes). The studies came into being through the interest of an orthopaedic surgeon, Norman Capener, who treated Hepworth's daughter Sarah for osteomyelitis in 1944: he had an eye for avant-garde art and purchased some of Hepworth's work at a time when life was difficult for her. In 1947, he invited her to observe an operation, sensing that her growing involvement with the structure of the body might find expression in a new work. Despite initial misgivings—his suggestion initially seemed to her "a grim idea"—she consented, visiting a number of hospitals in Exeter and London with a sterilised sketchpad and pencil. Over the next few years she made eighty drawings, working them up with a mixture of pastel, ink, chalk, oil and graphite on board, in some cases scoring the surface of the work with a razor blade to give it an urgent *sgraffito* quality. These are surface works: she never allows us to see the interior of the body, and there is no blood anywhere in her studies. Her drawings are decidedly not anatomical demonstrations. In 1953, she was even invited to lecture on "The artist's view of surgery", in which she made much of the similarities between the tasks of the surgeon and sculptor, especially when the surgeon was orthopaedic and wielding a hammer and chisel. She was able to make a group of doctors audience to their own performance.

You can sense the "sacrality" of the space around the masked anonymous surgeons, and the hallowed and even hushed zone of what must not be touched other than by those properly qualified and duly scrubbed up. The artist herself said that she was captivated, from the moment she entered the theatre, by "the extraordinary beauty of purpose and coordination between human beings all dedicated to the saving of life, and the way that unity of idea and purpose dictated a perfection of concentration, movement, and gesture." It was surely the case that the poise of the surgical staff induced a feeling of grace that came close to what she had been seeking in her own abstracts.

In the strip mines

In his cabaret-apocalypse *The Last Days of Mankind* (1915–1922), a satirical indictment of war with hundreds of scenes and a cast in the hundreds too, Karl Kraus wrote about one of the most sinister oxymorons of all—"human material," the Prussian general staff term for the men who were written off as spent forces on the fields of Flanders and Verdun.

The fact that every corporation and ministry now employs the analogous terms "human resources" or "human capital" without batting an eyelid suggests that R. G. Collingwood was right when he wrote that the Great War was "an unprecedented triumph for natural science" as well as "an unprecedented disgrace to the human intellect."

The advent of digital technologies at the turn of the millennium has advanced the process a degree further: we are now "human natural resources" for the owners of surveillance capital, who are conducting massive behavioural data mining operations on an agglomerated, interlinked and largely complaisant substrate.

Exiled from the implications of our own actions, held hostage in a state of ignorance: this is the shame of the colonised. We are, as Shoshana Zuboff says, "the native peoples now whose claims to self-determination have vanished from the maps of our own experience."

The hole and the whole

If philosophy is still to be seen in terms of Plato's cave, then tuberculosis—the cavitating disease—really ought to be regarded as the disease of thinkers and sceptics, not of artists and sensitive souls. Thomas Mann was inspired in making the chief character of *The Magic Mountain* a feckless young man, who decides to stay in the somnambulant atmosphere of the sanatorium in order to become a prig with a talent for illness. "Contemplation, retreat—there's something to it. One could say that we live at a rather high level of retreat from the world up here…". The engineer Castorp decides his task is to go *into* the cave and learn what it is to be a philosopher from the inside out. Not views but projections: such is the radiographic lesson life teaches him.

As the French doctor and writer Jean Reverzy wrote: "The revelation of the organs holds the same illusion as a shadow projected on a wall or a photograph taken from an unusual angle or the radioscopic image of a body: it is the disappointing recognition of a noble wish for knowledge and penetration that will never be satisfied."

That could be the definition of the magic mountain itself: a looming fabled place that retreats even as you approach it.

Saddle up

The saddle is, geometrically and topologically speaking, a complex and fascinating structure. It is a hyperbolic paraboloid, and therefore a structure to which the postulates of Euclidean geometry no longer apply. That was one of the great shocks for nineteenth-century mathematics: there was another kind of space available to geometers once the ancient prejudice about "parallel" lines had been ditched. The discovery of hyperbolic space by the Hungarian János Bolyai and the Russian Nicholai Lobatchevski in the 1820s was the beginning of what is now called non-Euclidean geometry. The difficulty for mathematicians, who were all male, was to discern a physical surface on which such a structure might be realised. It was only at the end of the twentieth century that Daina Taimina, a mathematician at Cornell University, suggested that crochet knitting provided some of the hyperbolic planes which could be observed in natural shapes such as lettuces and coral reefs.

Being a writer of parables, I feel instinctively drawn towards such an extravagantly hyperbolic dimension.

Recently I read Pascal Quignard's *Les desarçonnés*, the seventh volume of his Last Kingdom series, and yet another book in which he combines aphorism, philosophical excursus, observation and novelistic fragment. His book is a meditation on what it means to fall, specifically to fall out of the saddle. For that is the meaning of the verb *desarçonner*: to be unseated from the arçon, an old French word for the saddle tree. Trees and forests have supplied humans with primordial metaphors for notions of continuity and structure: there is the Tree of Life, and also the family tree; and there is the saddle tree, which at one point in human history, fastened securely between a horse's withers and croup, offered a man a seat as high as he could get in the world. Now, in an age when everyone is a pedestrian (or cocooned in his car), the attitude of a man on a high horse has come to seem slightly ridiculous.

Nevertheless, Montaigne wrote that if he were able to choose, he would "prefer to die in the saddle rather than in [his] bed, away from home and far from his folk" ("On Vanity"). He had several experiences during his life of falling from his horse, one of them almost fatal. Quignard—no doubt thinking of Saul on the road to Damascus and his conversion into Paul—is fascinated by the central role played by this experience of falling from a horse: he offers the expression *être desarçonné* as a humbler synonym for the experience of depression.

The philosopher Friedrich Nietzsche, who rode at a gallop in his writings and even imagined he was a centaur bestriding literature and philosophy, saw a painting of a horse by Vincent van Dyck that made him happy, but lost his mind when he witnessed the actual misery of a maltreated drayhorse in a Turin street and tried to prevent its owner from lashing it again. He had been saddled by his own imperious philosophy.

A DREAM OF MOIST MARBLE

The limb I was holding was cold and heavy and sweaty. I tried and tried, but to my alarm couldn't locate the radial pulse, not even the threadiest of beats. How was I going to take a sample for blood gases? Then I realised I was examining a marble statue by Praxiteles or one of his epigoni.

It must be true then that the old gods are dead, for the allure of the body was ancient divinity in its entirety.

THE FOLLOW-UP

"Offer counsel only to someone you don't expect to see again." A piece of advice that won't help you much if you're a general practitioner in the United Kingdom.

A DIVORCE

The French philosopher François Dagognet makes the distinction, in an interview (in the chapbook *Pour une philosophie de la maladie*), between "un médecin bon" and "un bon médecin"—in other words, a good doctor (in the moral sense) and an effective doctor (in the technical sense). He was picking up a discussion as old as Plato's *Republic*: the term "good" is unproblematic as a modifier of all kinds of different activities but becomes problematic when applied to aspects of social life—notably how we are to live together in the "good society"—that are not implicit in a practice. What the patient with a serious disease wants in the first instance is to be cured, if possible, not to be the recipient of pity or even kindness (though they may help)—and therefore requires the services of an effective doctor. Galen, the famous second-century Roman doctor from Pergamum, was just such an effective doctor, never once in his voluminous writings expressing any emotion, whether positive or negative, for a patient. Lacking sympathy, however, the effective doctor can have no idea of what the illness represents in the life of his patient.

The practical outcome of this situation is that the patient may often have a double disease and need to be treated twice. The patient's lived experience and not just his body is subject to the Cartesian divide. This is apparent with many cancer patients who, once they have been through the existential drama of surgery feel so brutalized or misunderstood that they attend naturopaths or take homeopathic medicines or visit a psychotherapist for the first time in their lives.

[Dagognet's distinction also applies, with altered freight, to the terms "une femme sage" and "une sage femme": the former is a prudent woman and the second a midwife: age and experience attach to both, although I've known some young midwives who were "wise" only in the street sense.]

Gentle and honest man

Dr Johnson was notably uncomfortable about his academic title, and made it clear to his correspondents that he preferred to be thought just an ordinary bloke—"un gentilhomme comme un autre." A similar tribal distinction is still observed with British surgeons, whose correct title is Mr and not Dr, presumably because it took them the best part of the late eighteenth- and early nineteenth-centuries to shake off the down-and-dirty reputation that clung to their origins as barber-surgeons: they wanted to be seen primarily as gentlemen rather than doctors (whose status in the early nineteenth century wasn't above reproach either).

Dr Johnson could equally have had in mind that famous entry by the French philosopher Blaise Pascal when he writes about his displeasure with those who wear their specialisations like uniforms. He much prefers those "universal people" who blend in with the crowd but are good when problems crop up, being able to deploy unsuspected talents when called upon by others. "We ought not to say of them either 'he is a mathematician' or 'he is a preacher'," writes Pascal, "but 'he is an *honnête homme*.' Only this universal quality pleases me."

It is an excellence that presumably extends to other domains too.

Pity as a fallacy

It could be the medical humanities movement is really little more than a glorified *argumentum ad misericordiam*—that is, an appeal to pity in order to improve either the standing of doctors now that the population in general has become mightily suspicious of anyone who seeks to do good, or an attempt to capitalise on the victim status that is so often sought these days when things go wrong.

An argument that turns on an appeal to pity is a fallacy, as are many consequentalist arguments, although the red herring of desirability may not necessarily invalidate the invited conclusion or indeed the facts as they stand.

Being in the papers

Nowadays it is assumed to be such an obvious pairing that nobody even sees fit to justify the unholy hybrid that now goes by the name "medical humanities". Yet we only have to go back to Flaubert's era, the mid-nineteenth century, to find that the notion of a physician-writer—a figure who enjoys a special cachet in our day as the exponent of a kind of clinical realism or expert in the social emotions—was actually an *insult*. Flaubert's great novel *Madame Bovary* was regarded as being a particularly dangerous kind of "physiological novel", from which women, in particular, had to be protected. Some of its critics suggested that it was time to stop talking of literature—"we are in a dissection room, and we have just read an autopsy report" (Alfred Nettement). Another critic suggested Flaubert was a "surgeon who was mistaken about his vocation" (Gustave Merlet). It was no distinction at all to be a physician who used his pen to write novels, and the collocation was even tainted with disrepute.

This attitude persisted until well into the 1970s, as Oliver Sacks reminds us in his autobiography *On the Move*. His father once barged into his bedroom, clutching that day's London *Times* in his hands, to tell his son aghast that he was "in the papers."

Although the article in question was actually a commendatory review of his first book *Migraine*, for his doctor-father, it was the last place he wanted to see his son's name, since writing by physicians for a popular audience was, in those days, considered to be a lapse of taste at best and a breach of ethics at worst—"I had committed a grave impropriety, if not a criminal folly, by being in the papers."

Perhaps we are in the confines of a different kind of consolatory morality when literature *has* to be good for you. But Flaubert is there to remind us: "there is no literature of good intentions: style is everything."

A FORTUNATE STATE

It seems strange that political commentators never underline the parallels between the pioneer settlers in Palestine and subsequent kibbutz movement, and the foundation of the National Health Service in the UK. Not only were the movements contemporaneous, they shared the same vision of a better and more cohesive society being created by the communal efforts of those with the means and the inclination to work for the good of those less fortunate or in need.

From about 1950 to 1980 general practitioners in the UK could almost afford to be indifferent to the claims of money and commercialism generally: their livelihood was guaranteed. And this freedom allowed the most complete development anywhere of the humane tradition in medicine, which embraced a form of clinical analysis based on multiple paradigms, a scientist's ability to interpret statistical data, a sensitivity to the patient's social life and the complexity of moral issues, and the deep solidarity with patients that John Berger captured in his description of the life of the rural practitioner Dr John Sassall in *A Fortunate Man*. "Sassall has to a large extent liberated himself and the image of himself in the eyes of his patients from the conventions of social etiquette. He had done this by becoming unconventional. Yet the unconventional doctor is a traditional figure."

Luminescence

The Buddha wears his neocortex on the outside of his head, to judge from the gold light shimmering around his head in some depictions. According to the American poet Robert Bly, meditating Tibetan monks in the thirteenth century were able to read in the dark by the light emanating from their own bodies. Well, I know the story of miners in Scotland allegedly being able to read down the mines of Fife—the air being too poor for their tallow lamps—by the phosphorescent light given off by herring scraps, but these fishy stories were most certainly long dead before they started giving off their own peculair marsh light. "Better an *ignis fatuus* / Than no *illume* at all", as the marvellous Emily Dickinson wrote.

When the fire flickers

It seems to have been Graham Greene who first gave currency to the notion of "burn out" in his 1960 novel *A Burnt-out Case*, in which the doctor running a leper colony in the Congo establishes a parallel between his guest, the architect Querry, tired of his celebrity, and the leprosy cases whose disease could no longer continue to mutilate their physical substance because it had "burned itself out". A decade later, the remarkable psychiatrist Herbert Freudenberger (1926-1999), who started the free clinic movement and worked with substance abusers in New York at a time when there was little interest in and few institutions to care for such people, used the expression to describe those of his patients who had been physically and mentally crippled by the use of hard drugs: he subsequently used the expression metaphorically to describe his own feeling of complete lassitude one morning when he found himself unable to get out of bed. He was on to something (although he might have diagnosed himself simply as "overworked and exhausted"). It was his clinical textbook detailing the various "phases" of burn-out in 1980 which loosed the name into the public arena.

Religious history also provides a tributary of meaning: *acedia* or *accidia* was the indifference of the soul which had lost the love of God. It was a condition that could grip the most fervent monk, and was of course a deadly sin. In Helen Waddell's famous translation from the fourth-century Latin, *The Desert Fathers*, acedia was described as "tedium or perturbation of the heart... akin to dejection and especially felt by wandering monks and solitaries, a persistent and obnoxious enemy to such as dwell in the desert, disturbing the monk especially about midday, like a fever mounting at a regular time... And so, some of the Fathers declare it to be the demon of noontide which is spoken of in the Ninety-first Psalm."

This remittent fever might have recurred at the hottest and brightest time of the day but it was marked by coldness. Glacial coldness. It was the sin of listlessness, of being turned away from the surroundings and indifferent towards others and the bright evidence of God's love; whereas in our mercantile civilisation of flux and liquefaction, burnout is an affliction of hotness, a disorder that affects people with naked ambition and the all-consuming desire to define themselves through their careers. "Intensity" is one of the most positive modern motive-words, a quality which describes the "peak state" sought in so many exploits from sport to sexuality.

But one day, having worked for weeks, months, perhaps years to meet targets in the company's strategy plan, an ambitious young employee is suddenly assailed by the realisation that her subjectivity is being exploited by a corporation hell-bent on creating profits for its shareholders above all else. A beautiful illusion collapses. And let us be frank: the more "burn-out" is discussed in the media the more acceptable it becomes. To be burned out distinguishes you as a person of refinement: it is a respectable diagnosis, implying that the sufferer has sacrificed her health for a higher cause than her own well-being—for the sake of work.

Le mal des croyants has reversed its polarity. Burning out is the sacrifice we bring that to the unholy modern trinity of mobility, instantaneity and manipulability.

The civil status of medical definitions

Psychopathology, as others have recognised, is the most extreme of the circular processes by which a psychiatric aberrancy is inferred from the antisocial behaviour of a person even while the mental anomaly is advanced to account for the same person's antisocial behaviour. The illness is the cause of the behaviour for which it is also the excuse.

Joining the others

Seleucus' seemingly cynical phrase at the famous decadent dinner with the nouveau riche Trimalchio in Petronius's novel of ancient Rome could so easily be updated to a night-club party in our era of wide boys and easy girls. Seleucus is lamenting the death of his friend Chrysanthus who—after going on a starvation diet on the recommendation of his doctors—"has gone to join the majority."

There follows a phrase in which Seleucus defines the true nature of the medical art—*Medicus enim nihil aliud est quam animi consolatio*—which Frederic Raphael translates in the same spirit: "After all, the doctors are there just to perk us up on the way out" (Satyricon 42).

Seleucus's maxim prompts a definition of the medical profession I hadn't thought of before: escort agency.

Grace time

When my wife used to do her district nursing rounds on the other side of the Rhine, in the Baden district known as the Ortenau, she carried a large black ring-binder folder in her car holding about a dozen laminates with bar-codes at the bottom of each page.

After every visit to a patient, she had to key in the patient's details, and relay information to a central databank about the procedure she had just performed by scanning the applicable bar-code with a hand-held scanner. And if this blatantly bureaucratic expedition of what was previously the most charitable of human acts wasn't enough of a shock for me, I discovered a stand-alone code on the last page: "menschliches Handeln"—a rough translation of which might be "humane acts." This was meant to cover time spent with the patient that couldn't be accounted for as a nursing procedure: asking patients about the weather or their grandchildren, for instance, or merely how they were feeling. It was limited to ten minutes.

But why was I so shocked? This is what Thatcherism did to the NHS in the 1980s—evacuating the concept of "public service" and "common good" in favour of an hourly payment rate determined under market conditions, and under contractual terms that allowed for advanced time-and-motion studies of every minute of a nurse's day. Each "item" of care was reconceptualised not in terms of its own intrinsic nature but as an auditable unit, which left no room for the fact that professional people did things for the patients because they cared for them, not because they expected to be paid for putting themselves out.

The purpose of this extreme functionalism is not to serve patients, but to provide data for managers to manipulate—as underscored by the fact that any questioning of the superstructure by those actually working on the ground is disallowed, and in fact may not even be expressible in the idiom of managerial legitimacy.

A REVELATION

During my period as a health development consultant in Sumatra I had to take shelter with colleagues in the staffroom of a community health centre one afternoon during a sudden tropical downpour. Since we were going to be doing an inspection of the site and noticing the empty waiting room I asked the chief doctor (raising my voice to make it heard against the throb and paradiddle of the rain on the roof) what the clinic's main problem was. "We don't have enough water," she replied, and didn't seem to register the blank stupidity of her answer. What she was really saying was that she wasn't interested enough in the welfare of the local people to use her influence with the local mayor to have some kind of simple capture and storage system built on the grounds or incur the additional moderate expense of having a gutter fitted to the roof. It was, after all, a property belonging to the district health authority.

Her attitude—which I ran into often enough in Indonesia among government-employed doctors who never earned enough to make it worthwhile for them to work in these clinics—betrayed almost Soviet-style assumptions about district government's lack of accountability as a provider of health services on the one hand, and a frank disdain for the poor on the other.

For the next half-hour in this ramshackle and decaying health clinic I tried to remember which poem Elizabeth Bishop had closed with these apposite lines:

> And never to have had to listen to rain
> so much like politician's speeches...

Carnifex

Joel Harrington's book on the sixteenth-century Nuremberg citizen Master Frantz Schmidt, who died in 1634 in a splendid town house and with a certificate from the Emperor confirming his burgher status, and for the life hereafter had the legend "physician" carved on his tombstone, suggests that behind the figure of the doctor-surgeon stands a more sinister one: the executioner.

In addition to treating more than 15 000 patients, according to his own account, Schmidt dispatched 228 persons by various methods including hanging, beheading and breaking on the wheel, not to mention less lethal but stigmatising procedures such as torturing, branding, amputation and flogging. These public executions had their element of spectacular excitement, the full severity of the law being acted out on a scaffold or stage in which the suffering of a condemned man provided a kind of gruesome theatre. But Schmidt lived in premodern times; the writers of the eighteenth century had yet to define the conditions for sympathy, itself a disconcertingly theatrical experience (as the title of that famous weekly *The Spectator* would suggest).

By contrast, the French "Royal Executioner", Charles-Henri Sanson (1739-1806), found the family business so distasteful he announced, as a young man, his intention to study medicine. He was, however, compelled to return to the trade in order to support other members of the family after his executioner father became incapacitated. Over the course of his life he dispatched no less than 2918 persons, including Louis XIV, and wrote an influential memorandum for the French Assembly on Dr Guillotin's new decapitating machine which ensured that the guillotine would go on to become the French nation's "humane" instrument of execution. The advent of the new killing device also raised his status from that of humble "bourreau" to "Monsieur de Paris".

Sanson sometimes dissected the bodies of those he executed. He also liked to cultivate his herb garden, had many musical friends, and was himself an excellent musician.

No place to hide

Medicine has been able to promote a therapeutic universality that exceeds the scope of any revealed religion. After all, nobody is a technophobe on the operating table, not even the Pope.

Split and double

She had recently undergone corneal lasering, she told me over dinner, and now one eye was calibrated for close reading and the other for long sight. Her brain had got used to it in a few weeks, she added blithely. My response was that this was the ophthalmological equivalent of the asymmetrical image of the face of Christ Pantokrator I had seen once in Saint Catherine's monastery in the Sinai, expressing His human and divine nature: one eye judges while the other forgives.

A similar duality is addressed in William Empson's recently discovered text on the Buddha, in which he claims that sculptors in the Mahayana tradition deployed facial asymmetry in order to display the dual aspect of the Bodhisattva—and indeed "to make the face more human". The Buddha's qualities—"complete repose or detachment" and "an active power to help the worshipper"—are fitted within the unity of the face, and the conflict between different kinds of attitude—the transcendentally remote and presently active, blindness and all-seeingness, self-sufficiency and universal charity—helps to create the mystery of the face. Of faces in general, it could be said.

This speculation is developed by a separate route in Julian Jaynes' *The Origin of Consciousness in the Breakdown of the Bicameral Mind*, in which he suggests that early humans heard god-voices in their heads telling them what to do. Iain McGilchrist's *The Master and the Emissary* offers an even more radically chambered vision of human being: he hypothesises that the formerly dominant right hemisphere (left face), which grasps reality as a living unified whole, has lost its ability to transmit these life-affirming messages to the left hemisphere (right face), which apprehends the world as mechanism.

Making good

"Jewish doctors are a kind of atonement for the crucifixion", wrote Joseph Roth in a letter. And for over a millennium, the best of them bore the forename Raphael, in honour of the archangel who was also the patron of healing (from the Hebrew *rapha*, to heal, and *el*, the element of divine being). Through the oppression of their own people they certainly knew all about *pathos*, in its literal sense of suffering and pain.

There is another explanation for the prominence of Jewish doctors in the middle ages, and especially during the great plagues when, as René Girard points out in *The Scapegoat*, there was no effective medicine at all. Jewish doctors were preferred because the power to heal was associated with the power to cause sickness. Show good will to the doctor, and he might spare you, that is to say: not infect you.

Translucidities

André Breton, the snobbish, dogmatic and autocratic leader of the Surrealist movement in 1930s' Paris, actually studied under the famous Joseph Babinski, Charcot's *chef de clinique* at the Salpêtrière and codifier of the famous plantar reflex known to all medical students.

According to the philosopher and medical historian François Dagognet, a whole generation of artists in that era sought to imitate the effect of X-rays, reading the interior of the cranium or the intimate details of body physiology behind its façade of clothes and blurred flesh. Surrealism was all about making a visible reality of the invisible, thereby redeeming one of the fundamental deficiencies of seeing.

In short, the surrealists wanted to enjoy the prestige of being radiologists without the inconvenience of losing their fingertips, as happened to many pioneers in the early days of *Roentgenologie*: X-rays had yet to acquire the reputation of being harmful at a distance in time. This was the fate of Blanche Wittmann, one of Charcot's most renowned *hystériques*, who, apparently cured, ended up working as an assistant in the Salpêtrière's new radiology laboratory: she died of cancer after undergoing several amputations.

"Whereas the first generation of X-ray explorers lived in a world in which science meant progress, today we are aware of the potentially lethal repercussions of exposure to radioactivity and are apprehensive about the delayed action of all kinds of invisible enemies from chemical pollution to dormant viruses to electromagnetic power lines," remarks Bettyan Holtzmann Kevles in her history of radiology *Naked to the Bone*. "The combination of invisibility and delayed reaction is still hard to grasp."

The curse of Venus

Most of the great Baghdad physicians were in no doubt: love is an illness, although they were willing to concede that "The opinions of the ancients diverged on the subject of this illness..." (Bakhtishu's *Medical Garden*).

Opinions of the wise doctors diverged about whether love was a feature of the reasonable or bestial soul, and whether it was due to an excess of appetite or an admixture of similitudes; but there is no divergence about its being *pathological*. They did not appear to consider that human significance could be generated from animal appetite, although there are plenty of hints of what being smitten meant to the three poets of the Abbasid Caliphate who appear in translation in the slim Penguin collection *Birds Through a Ceiling of Alabaster*.

From antiquity, the very notion of which persisted largely thanks to the preservation of the writings of Aristotle, to the beginnings of the second millennium in the great capital city of Islam, love often seems to have been experienced as an involuntary fact: Euripides' tragedy is about Aphrodite revenging herself on Hippolytus (who prefers to honour the god of the hunt Artemis) by smiting his stepmother Phaedra with the curse of love. The phrase "I love you" doesn't function in its modern sense, as a performative utterance; it is clear however that Phaedra is compelled to participate in the unfolding sense of what she already recognises in herself. That is the tragedy.

It takes the modern mind to make the phrase a promise that keeps a couple wed (if not necessarily married) as long as it can be repeated. The Baghdad physicians could not, it seems, imagine an age in which the verbal declaration of a felt emotion might be a confession of faith.

Illness as routine interrogation

The set of questions asked of a third party—when, what, how, how much, and for how long?—about a person who has taken a drug overdose and is showing all the signs of a toxidrome replicates the "hard facts" routine which cub reporters had to learn in the mid-twentieth century if they wanted a job with an American newspaper ("who, when, where, why, how?").

They also happen to be the so-called "minor" questions which, in Gilles Deleuze's philosophy, allow an Idea to be defined by its being differentiated from the other ideas immanent in the processes to which they have given form: an Idea (universal and transcendent) cannot be ascertained by asking the Socratic question "What is …?"

Preferred target

Friedrich Nietzsche, as is well known, hymned the praises of Dionysos, the god of the intoxicated will to live; his other diety, Apollo, had the power of clear articulate thought and disciplined insight. Nietzsche hoped they would live together in a kind of utopia of impulse and intellect. But Apollo, the god of medicine, is a more troubling character than Nietzsche ever let on.

Apollo, the god of light and the sun, truth and prophecy, medicine and music (and many other refined pursuits including archery), was also the god of plague. His arrows—the rays of the sun—could bring healing warmth, but they could also bring pestilence, and ultimately death. In the cities of Anatolia and Greece he was worshipped—apotropaically—in order to still the calamity he might let loose in that same place. Nietzsche turned him into a benign and serene god, but Homer perhaps had his truer measure when he called him "the most abominable" deity, an epithet which Plato—who like Nietzsche had invested in an intellectual project in honour of the god—considered a slander. (This ambiguity perhaps goes back at least as far as the ancient Babylonians, whose winged demon-god Pazuzu, one hand pointing up and one pointing down, was used as a charm to avert the wind-borne plagues he was thought to bring.)

The sun seems to be the connection between healing and disease, not least in its derivative form *fire*, which has always been considered the most effective means of purification. For that matter, the sun's rays are still understood as being both beneficial and harmful. Saint Sebastian became a popular cult in medieval times precisely because he was depicted as being stuck with arrows, and yet survived his martyrdom (to be martyred less glamorously a second time in an ancient WC). The hope was that his already tainted body would attract the roaming darts of disease and spare the congregation.

Although the real Sebastian was a middle-aged captain of the Praetorian Guard, he is invariably depicted by Renaissance artists as a handsome young man, often semi-nude: Vasari points out that his contorted cover-boy image and sweetly afflicted facial expression sometimes aroused inappropriate thoughts in church, particularly amongst female worshippers. (Emma Bovary even confesses in Flaubert's novel to having inappropriate tingling feelings—"de sensuels frémissements me couraient sur la peau"—about a painting of the "naked Man spread on the cross.")

It was a photograph of the famous chiaroscuro painting of the martyr naked except for a loincloth, arms bound behind his torso and gazing heavenwards by Guido Reni, a baroque painter of the Bologna school which goaded the young hero of one of Yukio Mishima's novels to his first orgasm. And Thomas Mann, in his famous novella *Death in Venice*, immediately saw the homoerotic connection with Apollo. The arrows of pestilence that claim the life of his composer-hero Aschenbach are the darts of desire. Fingers pointing inwards, as it were.

Added value

André Gide in his early symbolist work, *Paludes* (*Morasses*), wasn't impressed by notions of normality. Being healthy was simply a kind of mediocrity, where everything was in balance and nothing was hypertrophied. Idiosyncracy was the spectacular illness that made a man interesting. He has his character Valentin put it thus: "Now stop regarding *illness* as a lack; on the contrary it's a something added: a hunchback is a man plus his hump, and I'd rather that you regarded health as a lack of illness."

Lichtenberg, the gibbous German philosopher, would certainly have agreed.

Listen in

No other medical anecdotes offer the hard impress of the real like those in Miguel Torga's diaries, of which there were sixteen individual volumes—each one of them written during his long life as an ear, nose and throat specialist and general physician in the Trás-os-Montes region of northern Portugal. (Excerpts from them can be found, in translation, over twenty-four pages of my anthology *The Body in the Library*). But I've often wondered if Torga ever felt discomfited by the obligations of the Hippocratic Oath, which insists that "whatsoever in the course of practice you see or hear that ought never to be broadcast, you will not divulge." His recollections of his patients, some of whom must have been illiterate, strike me as being very close indeed to the bone and marrow of actual clinical encounters—exploitative and appreciative in equal measure. Hippocrates leaves the matter of gauging the force of the "ought" to the physician; yet it could never be said that Torga "betrays" his patients, since he respects their ordinary humanity and makes it manifestly clear that what they have told him—their confidences—have given him the courage to continue as their doctor.

After you

Now that Americans resort, more and more, when talking about the only reliable event in life (other than taxes), to that toe-curling euphemism "passing"—as in "he's passed" and don't even bother to add the postpositional particle "on" or "away", making it sound as if what they really want to say is "he's past" (as in tense), it comes as something of a relief to confront the plain unadorned fact of the matter, and no edulcoration. But only in British English—and for how much longer?

PRIVILEGES OF THE KITCHEN

In early modern times, the practical knowledge required to make concoctions of plants and herbs for therapeutic use was not distinguished from the instructions used to convey many other matters of fact. Recipes are now associated with lists of exotic ingredients, experiments in the kitchen and the moral exhortations of star chefs (especially at Christmas), but three or four centuries ago they provided instructions for experiments in metallurgy, painting, fireworks and gunnery as well as in the pharmacy. They were essential to the production and transfer of knowledge—that is towards openness, although the secrecy that often surrounded them was paradoxically an enticement and an invitation to enter a shared community of people "in the know". The recipe was a prescription for a subsequent "to do".

APOLLO AND MARSYAS

The archaic dream-master who really ought to strike terror into people is not wild, unkempt, amoral Dionysos but his half-brother, the coolly clinical Apollo—Apollo Medicus, god of halogen lamps, white coats and peremptory judgement.

It was Apollo's oracle at Delphi that was consulted for remedies to rid the city of the plague because it was he who, in his guise as god of pestilence, had brought the epidemic to the city in the first place. His essential doubleness is conveyed by the term *pharmakon*, which, significantly, may be pill or poison. Apollo's many epithets included Apotropaeus ("averter of evil") and confirm the impression that he was a god who was not to be invited, under any circumstances, into the house.

Ovid, in Book 6 of his *Metamorphoses*, retells the most savage myth of all in which Apollo in his guise as god of music hanged Marsyas on a pine tree and flayed him—"meticulously" as the Polish poet Zbigniew Herbert puts it—after the god turned out, in their famous contest, to be the better musician: he could sing and accompany himself on the lyre, expressive of the higher faculties, whereas Marsyas had only his rustic flute or pipe (*aulos*) on which to engross himself in making music. Marsyas' doodling on the pan-pipes was all immediacy and paroxysm: it was an improvisation, brilliant perhaps but somehow imprecise.

Ovid spares no detail in his description of Marsyas' punishment, as he slowly ends up *scarnificato*, stripped of all flesh: "Blood flowed everywhere, his nerves were exposed, unprotected, his vessels pulsed with no skin to cover them. It was possible to count his throbbing organs, and the chambers of the lungs, clearly visible within his thorax".

The "orgiastic flute", as Nietzsche calls it, stands not only for a grotesquely altered body image (in another myth Athena discarded the *aulos* after noticing that having to puff out her cheeks to play it ruined her looks) but a primitive sense of getting down and dirty. The fact that bags could be added to wind instruments to avoid the loss of facial composure, as when Nero played the pipes "by tucking a skin beneath his armpit, with a view to avoiding the reproach of Athena", only worsened the problem: what was this, an exteriorised lung or a distended stomach?

The belief in stringed instruments as "noble" and the pipes as "low" has persisted to this day. And modern anatomists have the perfect mythic backdrop for illustrating to their students how to acquire perfection in the instrumental art of inflicting the ultimate humiliation—stripping someone of his identity. "*I'll have your hide!*" as the saying goes.

Apollo, beneath white puffs of cloud, appears to be plying Marsyas' own bone flute as the flensing knife. His aesthetic is so pure and refined it hasn't the slightest appreciation of what it means to suffer.

An oxymoron

The first persons to come across the manuscript published by a London printer in 1642 as *Religio Medici* would have thought the terms of the title at odds with each other. Sir Thomas Browne—as complete a natural philosopher as it was possible to be in his day, with degrees and titles from Montpellier, Padua and Leyden—was at pains to reassure his readers he was a Christian in spite of "the generall scandal of my profession, the natural course of my studies, the indifferency of my behaviour, and discourse in matters of Religion." Medicine's origins were pagan, it was associated with Arabs and Jews, and having the gift of healing was often regarded as an occult art: those were the scandal of the profession. Browne's answer to his implicit words of self-criticism was to take the line that investigating the ways of nature would ultimately be a means of glorifying the Creator "through a devout and learned admiration."

Dr Adam will call you in

Nothing reminds us so strongly of the original onomastic power in the Garden of Eden when the Divine Creator brings the animals and fowls to Adam, "to see what he would call them", than the tendency to invent medical conditions and syndromes. What could be more reassuring for doctor and patient? You come to the surgery with a vague complaint of ill-defined pain, which has perhaps been lingering for months, even half forgotten at times, only for it to flare up again unbidden in the middle of the night; and you leave the consulting room in the knowledge that it now has a name, possibly even one with classical pretensions. Trochanteric bursitis, restless legs, irritable bowel syndrome, fibromyalgia (transliteration of symptoms into a Latin-Greek compound which simply means "pains in soft tissues and muscles") or the baroque Munchhausen's syndrome.

Many clinicians know such terms do not constitute an established diagnosis with a physical pathology; patients prefer not to. At least that is what John Berger surmises in his famous portrait of a GP, *A Fortunate Man*, having crammed up on Balint's *The Doctor, His Patient and the Illness*: "That is why patients are inordinately relieved when doctors give their complaint a name. The name may mean very little to them; they may understand nothing of what it signifies; but because it has a name, it has an independent existence from them. They can now struggle or complain *against* it. To have a complaint recognized, that is to say defined, limited and depersonalized, is to be made stronger." In other words, a disease with a name thinks it is already on the way to a cure.

F. G. Crookshank, a now forgotten philosopher of medicine, begs to demur. "In modern Medicine this tyranny of names is no less pernicious than is the modern form of scholastic realism. Diagnosis, which... should mean the finding out of all there is wrong with a particular patient and why, too often means in practice the formal and unctuous pronunciation of a Name that is deemed appropriate and absolves from the necessity of further investigation." It is hard to think of a more telling attack on the *Diagnostic and Statistical Manual of Mental Disorders*, which gets fatter with every new edition.

"'Diseases' are Platonic realities: universals *ante rem*", continued Crookshank. "This unavowed belief, which might be condoned were it frankly admitted, is an inheritance from Galen, and carried with it the corollary that our notions concerning this, that, or the other 'disease' are either absolutely right or absolutely wrong, and are not merely matters of mental convenience."

Already Immanuel Kant had warned against this habit. "Doctors believe that they have greatly benefited their patient when they give a name to his illness."

LIVING LIKE A GOD

Somebody on a French television programme—yet another talking-heads programme about books—made a nice distinction between what she called *le corps de souffrance* and *le corps de jouissance*: the former state of suffering was indisputably the lot of almost every human until the mid-twentieth century, while only those persons fortunate enough to be born in the developed West, at least since 1968, have had the inestimable privilege of being able to enjoy their bodies, so to speak. Prior to the modern era *jouissance* (an untranslatable French word which denotes the subjective consummation of a pleasure but also carries an older, juridical sense of legal entitlement or possession) was the privilege solely of the aristocratic class.

The speaker's distinction is one that has struck me as valid (enough to overcome my usual suspicion of the vacuousness of much French theorising). A vivid historical work about the nature of ordinary peasant or urban life in premodern society, e.g. Piero Camporesi's *Bread of Dreams*, suggests that if you were fortunate enough to make it through childhood, life was very likely to be—as Hobbes intimated—"poor, nasty, brutish, and short" (although it was most unlikely to be "solitary"), even inside a political economy. In so many respects we now enjoy the living arrangements of the classical gods. No human society has ever been provided with such levels of education, hygiene, leisure, general amenities and sexual indulgence. As it has been pointed out however, "one of the 'paradoxes of prosperity' is that people in rich countries don't realise how good things really are."

Circus acts

Medicine hasn't always been a closeted activity, with the physician sworn to uphold the confidentiality of the clinical encounter, something to which the French give great importance (recalling perhaps the intimate secrecy of the confessional).

In classical times, medicine was an *agon*—a competitive and public event at which an audience gathered to observe the skill (or otherwise) of physicians as they debated, demonstrated and dissected. Ancient sophistry had found a place in the clinical setting, and learned how to make a drama out of a crisis. The event might take place at the bedside, in which case a small group of select friends might be invited, or in a theatre, when an anatomical demonstration even began to resemble an unpleasant kind of circus act: Galen for instance would vivisect animals, disembowelling a monkey for instance, and taunting physicians in the audience by asking them to restore the intestines to the abdominal cavity. Only he had the requisite skill to do so, though he once confessed he didn't like the expression on the monkey's face when he cut open its belly.

Politics and madness

The French Revolution was regarded by its opponents as madness and mayhem unleashed on the earth. Edmund Burke, writing in 1790, suggested that its mass uprising had stripped the mind of the power of reason, and had left the French people in "an incomprehensible spirit of delirium and delusion." Philippe Pinel, superintendent of the vast asylum at the Bicêtre hospital in the south of Paris, drew up lists of forms of madness, the longest of which consisted of "Events Connected with the Revolution." Fear of the guillotine had reduced many people to "pusillanimity" and "dark despondency"; fear of random loss of family and property was just as coercive on the mind.

And yet the same Pinel, also in 1790, had observed the "salutary effects of the progress of liberty" and a general quickening of the national temper. The old rot was gone, and a new vigour and purpose was present "as though by some electric virtue." Everywhere he went he heard people exclaiming "I feel better since the revolution." It was an issue which would be debated throughout the nineteenth century, as France fluctuated between restoration and revolt. Bénédict-Augustin Morel, head of the Maréville asylum in Nancy, argued after the 1848 revolutions in his *Traité des maladies mentales* that political unrest and mass movements drew the isolated and solitary out of their private suffering and into the public domain.

Could it be that revolutions are perpetrated by very slightly mad people rather than the descendants of Rousseau's "new man"?

Lick and sniff

The old books say that tuberculosis has the odour of stale beer, yellow fever of a butcher's shop, and typhoid of freshly baked bread. The only disease I've ever diagnosed by smell was diabetes in a newly presenting patient who handed over a urine specimen for me to test in the surgery: it gave off the telltale smell of acetone, a by-product of the decomposition of acetoacetic acid. You can sometimes catch this smell on the breath of a patient—what the Portuguese doctor and novelist António Lobo Antunes describes as "the applesauce halitosis of a diabetic".

Warmth and comfort

Perhaps the most telling description of human society in the form we know it is the parable included by Arthur Schopenhauer in *Parerga and Paralipomena*: he writes about the dilemma faced by porcupines or hedgehogs ("Stachelschweine") in cold weather. His "company of porcupines" who "crowded themselves very close together one cold winter's day so as to benefit from one another's warmth and thereby prevent themselves from being frozen to death. But soon they perceived one another's quills, which induced them to separate again." And so on. The porcupines were "driven backwards and forward from one trouble to the other, until they found a mean distance at which they could most tolerably exist." In spite of good will, the parable suggests that intimacy cannot be entered upon without the risk of substantial mutual harm.

The hedgehog parable seems an instructive one for our era of demutualisation when so many of the associations and arrangements for a tolerable existence that sprang up in Schopenhauer's lifetime are being disbanded or having to modify their fiscal status.

It also suggests that Schopenhauer deserves to be ranked with Hobbes as a philosopher who thought human beings were essentially asocial by nature, and had to be forced into fellowship.

Facing them stand the moral sense philosophers, who left us workable theories of political economy and were convinced of our essential sociability. Many of them were from eighteenth-century Scotland, a most convivial nation.

Which makes me think of Randall Jarrell's brilliant quip: "soon we shall know everything the eighteenth century didn't know, and nothing it did, and it will be hard to live with us," which is a kind of porcupine spine itself.

Samaritan logic

He explained to me how socialism (what in the USA is called "liberal thinking") becomes decadent. An act of compassion is effective only when it is *unanticipated* by its recipient. Once the "gift" becomes enshrined as an act of the state, receipted by anticipation and considered thereafter an entitlement, it perverts the supposition that the underlying point of welfare is to help its recipient return to productive life in our all-encompassing market system. Both giver and receiver remain mired in the depressive features of an impersonal modern mechanism which was first devised to remedy extreme poverty.

That at least was how welfare was supposed to function in the market economy of the United States, far from any kind of threat of invasion or military campaign on its own soil. It occurred to me that there was a much darker interpretation of welfare in Europe: it was about preparing for war, at least in Bismarck's developing Germany. And in Britain, the National Health Service was born, at least in part, out of a widespread sentiment of solidarity: the camp-bed situation of being bombed together. But if the camps had been put up by the Scouts of the British Empire, the beds had been made by the secular metaphysics that the idealist philosopher T.H. Green (1836-1882)—only the most prominent of a whole line of ethical socialists—developed out of his reading of Hegel.

My hands are my heart

Gabriel Orozco's artwork *Mis manos son mi corazón* (1991) offers a set of two frontal photographs of the bare-chested artist: the first depicts him squeezing his hands around a soft lump of clay, the second with his hands open and holding the resulting heart-shaped form towards the viewer. As well as being an allegory of the most archetypal creative act of all, the second photograph of "My Hands are my Heart" recalls the seventeenth-century Catholic mystic tradition of the Sacred Heart—Jesus' physical, bleeding heart as a representation of His love for humankind.

Jesus's last words on the cross were a quote from Hebrew scripture, the opening of Psalm 22. One of the later lines of that austerely beautiful song of abandonment runs thus: "My heart is like wax; it is melted in the midst of my bowels".

To a medical eye, however, the striated terracotta cast held inside Orozco's hands looks much more like the sacrum, the large triangular bone at the bottom of the spine, which also protects the organs of procreation in the pelvic cavity and anchors the hip bones. It is the bone that bears the mark of our passage from youth to adulthood, since the five bones which constitute it (like the fingermarks in the artist's clay) usually fuse into one solid structure around age 26.

My Hands are my Sacrum as a votary image wouldn't be misplaced either: its name derives from the Latin "sacer" and in German (and the Slavic languages) it is still called "the cross". Suffering lumbago or back pain in those cultures brings you, philologically at least, to a plane where you can identify with the woes of the Redeemer.

What we know

Happiness goes underground, lives clandestinely and talks an obscure classical language in a mercantile society completely given over to calculation. Dante tells us that joy, happiness and love are *gratuities*. That must be why nobody wants to go to paradise now—it has no entrance fee. Modern people would rather roil and toil in hell, having built it themselves.

Bare plots

Close reading—the practice associated with the movement known as New Criticism—isn't the only way to approach a piece of writing. New Historicism opts for placing literary works in their historical and social context, and is associated with Marxism and more recently the French philosopher Michel Foucault.

Both approaches find a parallel in the clinical setting. But if what critics do is analytical, what doctors do is often *anatomical*: they cut a long story short, parse it in ingenious, abrupt and sometimes violent ways in order to reduce it to its bare plot lines: the solid vertebrae that hold up the fleshy superstructure.

The enterprising Russian theorist Viktor Shklovsky was a specialist of this method. In his book *Energy of Delusion*, he suggests that some of the stories of Chekhov, who was hardly a longwinded writer although he did sometimes meander, could be glossed in skeletal form. The man in his story "An Avenger" tries to come to terms, or reason with, the indignity of his being cuckolded, and enters a general hardware store with the express intent of purchasing a firearm. Deciding a firearm would be a tool too dangerous for a man in his unsteady frame of mind, he saves face by purchasing a birdcatching net although he doesn't have a clue about ornithology. This is how Shklovksy strips the story down to its essential dynamics, and takes the scales off our eyes:

> "He wants to kill his wife.
> He goes to buy a pistol.
> They offer him a variety of pistols.
> But then he begins to think.
> Kill her?
> Or maybe it's better to kill himself?
> Or maybe kill both of them?
> But he starts talking to the seller.

> Then he doesn't know how to leave the store.
> As a result he ends up buying a net for catching birds
>   that he doesn't need."

In Shklovsky's words, what an apparently realist story offers, once even the muscle flaps of development have been excised, is a plot that turns on "the negation of the ordinary through the ordinary." This kind of unadorned, clipped, defamiliarised idiom is reminiscent of some contemporary writers: the American Lydia Davis specialises in such kinks in the surface of the real. Her stories are anomalous non-events. The question is whether we can make anything of them.

WORK AND LEISURE

The French suspicion of British general practice and what they see as its control by the state stems from a vestigial remembrance of what the expression *ars liberalis* entails: liberal practice is work that is meaningful in itself. John Henry Newman was clear enough about the concept: "that alone is liberal knowledge which stands on its own pretensions, which is independent of sequel, refuses to be informed by any end." British doctors, in the eyes of their colleagues across the Channel, abandoned this historical form of guild practice and opted for *artes serviles*, i.e. chose to work in a way which, in the older sense of the term, is utilitarian: servile work is always work for a purpose, even if it is sacrificed for an idol called society. Yet the notion of a human activity that might be meaningful in itself died out a long time ago or became quaint, like writing poetry. For modern people even leisure has to be purposeful. That is one reason why the adjective "otiose"—from the Latin word "otiosus," meaning leisure—has acquired a pejorative slant in English.

(There are probably two other vestigial traditions at work in the French attitude: the old French tradition of anarchism, which has periodically—and paradoxically—attempted to organise itself into a political force, as in the twentieth-century movement known as

Unanimism, and that old Platonic contempt for the "banausic", as defined in the *Symposium*, where Plato redeploys the aristocratic contempt for manual labour to define the person who is not inspired by the daemon: only the daemonic man—the philosopher—is the truly wise person, an elitism which persists to this day.)

But the French are surely the more deceived. For doctors in both countries have since the end of World War II been working within the framework of social security systems that are bankrolled and controlled by the state. It's just that the French are more romantically defensive about their individualism. In France you're not entitled to intervene in somebody else's life, even those of close relatives, unless they explicitly ask you to; in the United Kingdom, other people invariably try to help you unless you tell them you don't want assistance. They attend to the neighbour's business before their own, as it were.

A LOST CAUSE

John Ruskin resigned from Oxford in 1885 during his second term there as its first Professor of Art when the University voted to allow the practice of vivisection in its laboratories. His idea of science was akin to Goethe's: it ought to allow for an understanding of the "beauty of the creatures subject to your own human life" (*The Eagle's Nest*, 1872).

FALLEN ARCHES

Hans Castorp, the hero of Thomas Mann's *The Magic Mountain*, puts his hand on a radiographic plate and has a premonition of his own death when he sees its bony structure outlined before him. Many children in the USA and Europe born between 1920 and 1960 had the experience of seeing not their hands but their feet in negative. This social phenomenon was a spin-off of American enthusiasm for the Coolidge tube, an X-ray tube with an improved cathode which had been installed in the Army's portable radiography units: these allowed reasonable penetration and visualisation of deeper tissues.

Adapted for commercial use, these devices found a ready market in the shoe industry. Shoe-fitting fluoroscopes, called the Foot-O-Scope by the Americans and the Pedoscope by the British, were installed in outlets across both countries. Children would ascend the steps, insert their freshly shod feet in the aperture at the bottom of the machine, press the button and marvel through a viewing porthole fitted at the top at their ghostly wriggling toes. Two other portholes at the side allowed the parent and shop assistant to determine whether the feet fitted the shoes. It was of course a gimmick, a trivial use for such a valuable technology, since the information the fluoroscopes provided could just as well have been provided by old-fashioned ways of measuring the feet. The dangers of unnecessary exposure to radiation were finally revealed in 1949, after which their use was phased out; although I can personally remember putting my foot in just such a machine in Clark's shoe shop in the south-side of Glasgow as a small boy, circa 1967. The machines surely had another role. They encouraged popular acceptance of a high-tech method that could "see" beyond the skin barrier, and whispered to parents and children alike that science was there to help—at least to make sure better-fitting shoes lasted longer.

Furor therapeuticus

"Acharnement thérapeutique": this common French phrase is difficult to translate. I have seen it translated as "therapeutic obstinacy" or "therapeutic zealotry", though neither term is quite right. It is defined by the dictionary as "prolonged and futile health care, of no benefit to the patient." One might quibble about whether the care need be "prolonged": one related idiomatic English expression—the ironic command "Please, no heroic measures!"—hints that what counts is a matter of scale rather than extension in time. A relentless, overblown futility is certainly part of the picture: that is why "acharnement" is often followed by an "escalade" (even more frantic treatment).

Often, "acharnment thérapeutique" is nimbly translated as "overtreatment"—presumably by analogy with that bureaucratic obscenity of the nuclear age, "overkill." There's nothing especially modern about "acharnement" though. Littré's famous dictionary points out that the word's origins lie deep in animality: "action of an animal determined to hold fast to the flesh it is devouring, to fight tooth and nail." It is rooted in the Latin "carnis" (of the flesh), and it seems to have entered everyday French as a specialist import word from hunting and falconry: "acharnement" referred to the baiting of a trap. It therefore indicates a kind of doggedness, or even brute mindlessness: that is why the word "acharnement" also turns up when the media have a feeding frenzy: everybody is in pursuit of the same story. Anybody subjected to that kind of attention is bound to feel hounded. "Ils s'approchent pour la curée"—then they move in for the kill, another hunting term. (At such moments the media are far closer to blood sports than they are to the polite vapidity of the term "communication".)

It's disconcerting to come across a deep intuition about the buried primitiveness of a seemingly mundane term in a writer from another language altogether—and one that doesn't have a medieval equivalent of the French expression. In a letter to his friend Max Brod at the end of April 1921, in which he reveals his definitive diagnosis (and severely limited prognosis) as a case of advanced and worsening pulmonary tuberculosis, Franz Kafka catches the spoor of the hunt. "Es gibt nur eine Krankheit, nicht mehr, und diese eine Krankheit wird von der Medicin blindlings gejagt wie ein Tier durch endlose Wälder." [There's only one disease, no more than that, and Medicine blindly hunts this one disease like an animal through endless forests.]

Alexandre Kojève predicted in his once influential reading of Hegel that when history ends—and along with it philosophy—it will not be a catastrophe: humans will become animals of a higher sort, i.e. contented creatures who live in harmony with nature and "react by conditioned reflexes to vocal signals or sign 'language'." But the flesh is always likely to dog our spirits; and if life is regarded purely as a biological phenomenon we may well invite the attentions of that other animal term that is so characteristic of French discourse: "bêtise"—as if when our technical sophistication reaches an apex it rediscovers something in us that snarls at intelligence.

Diagnosis and treatment

I discovered the Latin expression "ex juvantibus" only recently. It means "from that which helps" and alludes to a medical pitfall in which a treatment is substituted for a working diagnosis. In fact, the empirical response to a treatment may be a way of confirming a mooted diagnosis; on the other hand it is quite common these days to find people taking multiple medications on the assumption that all of them are helping, without anybody asking why they should be taking so many in the first place.

Trapped birds

Most medical students, and I was no exception, are confused by the terms used to describe the sounds heard on listening to the lungs with a stethoscope, the act doctors like to call *auscultation*: are "rales" the same as rhonchi or rattles, and when can you talk about "crepitations"? Back in 1977, the American Thoracic Society and College of Chest Physicians attempted to standardise the nomenclature, and suggested using the term "crackles". However, the older terms are still used.

The confusion, I discovered, goes back to the translation of René Laënnec's book *De l'auscultation médiate* by John Forbes, a year after its publication in France in 1819: he retained the word "rale" to denote "all the noises produced by the passage of the air, during the act of respiration, through the fluids in the bronchi or the lungs". This important text set out a systematic method for diagnosing diseases of the heart and lungs based on the use of the stethoscope, a device which Laënnec had developed and used at the Hôpital Necker in Paris. Initially a cylinder made of paper and then wood, Laënnec realised that the stethoscope amplified not just the sounds of the heart but also the various sounds made by air travelling through the airways. The stethoscope obliged doctors to examine their patients methodically, but also kept them at a hygienic distance; earlier clinicians (if they examined their patients at all) had simply applied their ear to a patient's chest.

The first thing that strikes the reader, when Laënnec attempts to distinguish between the various "râles" he could hear in diseased lungs, are his attempts at systematic description. He distinguished four types of rales: moist rales ("crépitations"), mucous or gurgling rales, dry sonorous rales and dry high-pitched or whistling rales. Attempting to describe the third and four types more precisely, he compared them respectively to a dovelike moan or cooing ("au roucoulement de la tourterelle") and to the piping of small birds ("au cri des petits oiseaux"). He was using natural analogies to distinguish subtle tonal differences in these sounds; they are not meant to conjure up an aviary though.

Evocation in a literary work operates on quite different principles. In some ways the most bravura form of evocation in literature is Hemingway's: an entire experience or scene is suggested with greatest economy of means. The reader's imagination fills the gaps. A scientific writer like Laënnec needs just as much skill as a creative one, but has to rein in the imagination of his (professional) readers as much as he spurs it on. Those readers are clinicians who, by dint of listening to chests on a daily basis, already possess "keen" ears, a kind of exquisite auditory sensitivity that makes it possible for them to perceive sounds and tones imperceptible to untrained listeners.

That the imagination is difficult to harness is suggested by Laënnec's patients, who took umbrage when he and his interns started using the word "râle" to describe their lung symptoms. They associated it with the "râle de la mort", the death rattle or sounds made by people about to die who can no longer clear secretions from their airways (Laënnec's second category). So out of a sense of delicacy, at the bedside, he avoided using the word "râle" and spoke of a "rhonchus", the Latin word for a snore. This was not understood by Forbes; hence the confusion in the English terminology.

A HAGIOGRAPHY

Even now, it is still possible to find evidence of saintliness in medicine. I saw evidence of it once, in outback Australia, when I was told about an entire mining town—a decade or two before I went there to work for a year—turning out for the funeral of a paediatrician who died relatively young, having given up a comfortable career in Sydney or Adelaide to come and work in what Australians regard as the sticks. He had made it his mission in life to alleviate their suffering, in particular the suffering of their children, whatever the cost to himself; and the cost in the end was his own life, which suited nobody. Those he had treated even if they weren't religious recognised an act of true devotion; and remembered him long enough in their hagiography of significant locals for me to hear about it.

The story made me think of Benassis, the doctor-hero of Balzac's novel *Le médecin du campagne* (*The Country Doctor*) whose cortege in the foothills of the French Alps is attended by 5000 people, every one of whom kneel as it passes. Or the account in one of his biographies of the local people of Rutherford, NJ, turning out with their families for William Carlos Williams' funeral in 1963. It was the hard-working local doctor they had come to praise, not the ground-breaking modernist poet whose work they never read.

ETHICS OF PERFECTIBILITY

So many nineteenth-century (and even quite a few twentieth-century) British writers seemed convinced of "the growing good of the world": Charles Darwin for one, and George Eliot for another, who wrote in *Middlemarch* that it was "partly dependent on unhistoric acts". By contrast, the German philosopher Max Scheler came to the conclusion, after being shaken to the core by the passions released in him by the Great War, that a world run on the principles of "fellow feeling" must include the negative emotions as much as the positive: *schadenfreude* as much as rejoicing at another's *largesse*. It was only after that terrible war that Europeans realised just how overconfident nineteenth-century sociology had been, both about itself and about progress in the general culture, which it understood as being freed from faith and brought into the clarity of analysis. "Progress," according to Herbert Spencer, "is not an accident, but a necessity, surely must evil and immorality disappear; surely must men become perfect." (*Social Statics*, 1892).

Darwin—Scheler notes—attributes increasing sociability with fellow-feelings solely of the positive kind. "This leads him to the fundamentally erroneous belief that 'social development' as such is in some sense a condition of moral *progress* and a source of *positive* moral energy."

Similarly, we still believe with blind optimism that everything "has a solution" although recent history has shown that final solutions can be very sinister indeed.

An immortal bag of wind

For two months, Thomas de Quincey tells us in *Confessions of an English Opium-Eater*, he suffered severe headaches, though his head had been a part of his body so free of physical weakness he had believed, as Horace Walpole used to say of his stomach, "that it seemed likely to survive the rest of [his] person."

Onion juice

Vincent van Gogh painted *Still Life with a Plate of Onions* in January 1889, shortly after returning to the "yellow house" on the Place Lamartine, Arles. He had been admitted to hospital just before Christmas in a critical state: having first brandished a razor at his friend and house-mate Paul Gauguin he used it to lop off the lower part of his own left ear. The still life (one of a hundred and ninety-four he painted in his career) shows his drawing board on a trestle between a bottle of white wine and a large green jug.

The American writer Guy Davenport, who has also written about this painting, says that its visual force attaches to "an utterly primitive and archaic feeling that a picture of food has some sustenance." Or could it be that Nature is a dead language that needs a painter to bring it to life? Variously arranged on the board are a pipe and shag tobacco in paper wrap, a bowl containing white onions, a candlestick and candle, a matchbox, sealing wax, a franked registered letter, upside-down in relation to the viewer, and a thick buff-coloured book. It is just possible to make out the title on the cover of the book: *Manuel annuaire de la Santé pour 1874 ou médicine et pharmacie domestiques contenant tous les renseignements théoriques et pratiques nécessaires pour savoir préparer et employer soi-même les médicaments par Frédéric-Vincent Raspail.* This was a hugely popular work, first published in 1845, whose full title reveals its purpose: it was a household pharmacy guide "containing all the theoretical and practical information" that would allow readers to prepare medications for their own use. Raspail was, like "l'pasteur Vincent", an instinctive, rather literal-minded democrat, who studied grasses because of "their humble, 'proletarian' place in the kingdom of nature." He believed in the healing properties of camphor, and his advocacy is largely responsible for its extensive use in the nineteenth century.

The volatile oils of *Allium cepa* have been used for much longer as a curative: I remember (to my shame) ridiculing my wife when she chopped up an onion, wrapped it in muslin and heated it gently in the microwave before wrapping it around our children's ears when they were suffering from glue ear, a problem that is the bane of small children owing to the slightly different morphology of the ear in early life as opposed to adulthood. The room smelt awful but by the morning their pain had gone. This homemade poultice would have been familiar to Hippocrates, who used syrup of onion as an expectorant and diuretic. Vincent van Gogh didn't need onions to make himself weep; he wanted them to cure him of his torments, though they certainly wouldn't restore his amputated earlobe.

And in the century following van Gogh's, it was discovered that onions, skinned and cut, could cover up the smell of the dead, as Günter Grass tells us in his controversial autobiography *Skinning the Onion* [*Beim Hauten des Zwiebels*]. For a day or two, perhaps.

Automatisms

Jean Epstein (1897-1953), film theorist and director of the silent film *Un cœur fidèle* (1923) which is famous for its many technically daring sequences including a kinetically adventurous fairground whirl, insisted on the buried connection between Charlie Chaplin—known to the French by his nickname "Charlot"—and the great neurologist Jean-Martin Charcot: "one has only to compare his gait to that of the psychiatric patients filmed at the Hôpital Salpêtrière between 1910 and 1912" to confirm that the celebrated comic, with his trademark lateral gait, was familiar with the spastic tics and marionette-like gait of neurological patients. Charcot, in fact, had been appointed head physician of the hospital in 1862, and became a celebrity himself by the mid-seventies, largely on account of his Tuesday lectures at which he exhibited his patients. Some of his students, who included Joseph Babinski, William James, Sigmund Freud and Gilles de la Tourette, became famous themselves, not to mention his patients, who came to widespread public notice through newspapers and journals.

Indeed, it has been said the angular, stuttering and frenetic style of early silent films owed as much to the many music hall performers who had adopted a new repertoire of movements and grimaces (even if they were unaware of their clinical origins) as to the visual flicker of the medium itself. Cabaret performers and comedians adopted puppet-like gaits and movements, and they were often the first performers recruited to serve in the new medium of cinema. Chaplin himself started out in the London music halls blending pathos and slapstick as a member of the mime troupe of Fred Karno's London Comedians, before touring the North American vaudeville circuit with the company and becoming famous for his ataxic "inebriate Swell" act. During his second tour, he was invited to join the New York Motion

Picture Company: that was the beginning of his other, famously mannered career in which intentionality proved to have, so to speak, a mind of its own.

The philosopher of the "élan vital", Henri Bergson, had in his book *Le Rire* (1900), defined the comic as "du mécanique plaqué sur du vivant" ["the living made to look mechanical"]— as the smooth continuity of everyday life being waylaid by jerky, machine-like, disruptive movements was intrinsically amusing. As the poet Charles Baudelaire had observed before him, there is something mechanically convulsive about a man who laughs. He has just fallen into the same kind of manhole that swallowed the clown he was laughing at only a moment before. This structural if not behavioural similarity is one reason why modern comedy is such a ticklish subject, and modern laughter often so nervous.

Be happy!

One of the wiser things written about the fabled state of happiness is John Stuart Mill's comment of 1873 that: "those only are happy (I thought) who have their minds fixed on some object other than their own happiness. Aiming thus at something else they find happiness along the way." In other words, happiness is a kind of phenomenon that is always out of focus; going in search of it is essentially a recipe for unhappiness; and all the theorising about how to be "in it" symptomatic of an age of confusion and even podsnappery.

That doesn't stop millions of self-medicating punters living its paradox, although wanting to preserve and protect happiness at all costs necessarily destroys any possibility of its lingering.

Hyperflexion

It is difficult to see how a good healer would be able to cultivate sympathy if he weren't keenly aware of the common lot. By observing suffering in other people, by relieving it sometimes, by forestalling it even, doctors imagine it can somehow be held at a distance. What we can't do is suffer in the place of others. We can attribute a sense to suffering, though the interpretation of its meaning may entail other, more subtle sufferings. As Kafka understood: "You can hold yourself back from the sufferings of the world, that is something you are free to do and it accords with your nature, but perhaps this very holding back is the one suffering that you could avoid." In other words, to seek to be relieved of suffering in one dimension is to be subject to it in another. We can feel the full force of this paradox when Dante's childhood friend Forese meets him in Purgatory and says "And not once only, as we circle round this road,/ Is our pain renewed: and though I say/ Pain it would be better to say solace…"

As sentient beings, it is impossible to live without suffering. If we wanted to suppress suffering, we would have to suppress life itself in order to be completely safe. Suffering makes people afraid. It makes some people so afraid they become doctors.

Kidneys and Cities

The association between the body and the state, specifically the city state, is an old one. John of Salisbury, the twelfth-century philosopher, is generally credited with making explicit the hierarchical image of a ruler sitting over society as its caput or head, with counsellors its heart, merchants its stomach, soldiers its hands and peasants its feet; he saw this image duplicated in the form of the city, with its cathedral, marketplace and houses of various quality and standing. Politics derives from the generic language of the body. Thus the city brings together people of various provenance, and subjects them to its politics.

Julian Green, the French writer of American origin who died as old as the twentieth century, once wrote a loving little tract about Paris, in which he discovered during the war that by looking at a map of the city for long enough it made him think of a brain. "Thinking about the capital all the time, I rebuilt it inside myself… I made the discovery that Paris was shaped like a human brain." He confessed that it had all to do with a split-head display that he had seen in an optician's window as a child.

The brain might seem the only appropriate organ for Paris, especially for an intellectual Parisian, but a steadier glance might have told him that he was manifestly projecting his own imagination over the stony city, magnificently spread out as it when seen from the butte de Montmartre. A more anatomically informed glance might have convinced him that Paris seen from the Montgolfier of the literary imagination betters fits the microscopic model of a kidney glomerulus nestling tidily inside its capsule with the grey-green river Seine—"the instinctive, unspoken part of our nature"—running through it. Come to think of it, most French cities have that encapsulated feeling, especially those that bear the traces of their walled, medieval fortifications: Paris's even gave rise to a famous saying: "le mur murant Paris rend Paris murmurant" (though it's more than a murmur that will come up to you these days if you walk out of old intramural Paris and over the six busy lanes of the orbital *périphérique*).

What do kidneys do? Their principal functions are to eliminate metabolic wastes containing nitrogen (which are toxic to the body) and regulate osmosis, thereby ensuring water and electrolyte balance in the body—what the philosopher famously called "*le milieu intérieur*". Enlightenment cities were obsessed with rediscovering the old Roman idea of the *urbs*, and the incessant circulation of water. Water running through a city was its life-blood. And it strikes me, sitting in Café Brant, looking over on to medieval Strasbourg, that nearly all French cities, having preserved their centres intact in spite of the ravages of the twentieth century, conform to the hydrostatic pattern of the kidney glomerulus. If Paris *intramuros* looks like a nephron, so too does Strasbourg, the orbital rondo of its urban life subtly regulated by the pressure gradient of the river Ill, which circumvents the old citadel. Thirteen hundred millilitres of blood pass through the glomeruli of the average kidney every minute; I'm not sure how much water flows through the Seine every minute but I do know that the Parisians drink the "same" water seven times.

Singapore, a city-state which doesn't have much water of its own, has developed a high-tech water recycling scheme using a dual membrane process to recycle domestic sewage to levels close to the quality of distilled water. Like the kidneys, these recycling plants use two membranes, one with larger holes to remove micro-organisms, while the second separates salt from water.

Walter Rathenau, the genial Weimar era politician and founder of the industrial giant AEG who was assassinated while serving as Foreign Minister of the Weimar Republic in 1922, imagined the modern metropolis (he meant Berlin) in one of his futurist books as a giant water heater with the plasma of subjectivity being pumped pneumatically through its sign systems and broadcasting centres—the same plasma which Ulrich, the main protagonist of Robert Musil's novel *The Man without Qualities* calls "universal nutritional fluid". The modern self recognises that it has some connection with the surrounding world but hasn't a clue what it might be.

Thinking of cities as kidneys reminded me of Montaigne who used to scrutinise his urine in the chamber pot every morning, to see whether he had passed the stones that caused him so much trouble. At least after his "attacks of the stone" he could pass the offending calculi; Sir Walter Scott lay sweating in agony for days, his colic so excruciating he asked for the New Testament to be read aloud to him. The pain was so awful some brave souls would go under the knife, a perilous procedure in that era; now we have lithotripsy, a form of ultrasound which pulverises the stone inside the body and allows it to be excreted as gravel. Having been present almost everywhere in Enlightenment literature, for instance in the novels of that earlier Scottish novelist Tobias Smollett, who was also a ship's surgeon, the kidney (along with many other body parts) was to vanish completely until James Joyce's *Ulysses*.

Many of the world's mega-cities have no or minimal schemes for waste management. Like vertebrates, planned cities evolved complex mechanisms in order to be chemically independent of their environments, and in order not to succumb like infusoria to gradual auto-intoxication. It might be simpler for unplanned cities to flush their waste straight out to sea, like a primitive fish that excretes nitrogen across its gills, but there is every chance the hypersea will come sludging back, and not as an allegory.

Only then might we notice that the entire human species is suffering under the regime of internal and external poisoning called *consumerism*.

His portrait

"Famoso Doctor Pareselsvs" reads the inscription on the copy of the painting by the Flemish painter Quentin Metsys or Massys, who is famous for his other medical study "Grotesque Old Woman", which hangs in the National Gallery in London: it inspired John Tenniel's depiction of the ugly duchess in *Alice in Wonderland*.

Philippus Theophrastus Aureolus Bombastus ab Hohenheim's better-known name (almost an epithet) was either a latinization of the homestead that was his birthplace in Switzerland or a bold claim to be considered on at least equal terms with the Roman encyclopaedist Aulus Cornelius Celsus, author of the compendious *De Medicina*. What we know of the quarrelsome Paracelsus (1493-1541) suggests the latter may be correct.

Trained in botany, metallurgy and mineralogy, his initial medical experience was as a surgeon in service to the armies of the Republic of Venice: in his *Die große Wundarzney*, he anticipated modern hygienic methods, recommending that wounds should above all be kept clean: "If you prevent infection, Nature will heal the wound all by herself." The physician who did nothing could seem to work wonders. This was evidently a challenge to conventional medical thinking of the time; once established as a physician in Basel, then a centre of humanism and bookmaking and where he treated the famous publisher Frobenius and encountered Erasmus, he lost no time in further antagonising the medical (and alchemical) establishment.

Banished from Basel he became an itinerant physician in the towns between the Upper Rhine and the headwaters of the Danube. Like Luther, he was openly defiant of instituted authority, ridiculed mere titles and maintained that only those who practised an art knew it: "The patients are your textbook, the sickbed is your study." He contradicted Galen's teachings of the prevailing doctrine of the "balance of humours". He recognized the distinctiveness of congenital illnesses, related specific diseases to occupations (tuberculosis and silicosis) or to mineral deficiencies (goitre and cretinism) and carefully described the symptoms of hysteria and other psychiatric manifestations. Carl Gustav Jung considered him a pioneer psychologist of the unconscious. Arthur Schnitzler wrote a one-act play about his abilities as hypnotist which calls into question the very stability of the mental life. Paracelsus advocated the use of chemical and minerals in medicine (humans being micro-versions of the great macrocosm of Nature), experimented on the human body and developed the tincture of opium known to the Victorians as laudanum. He even came close to imagining that disease might be due to external factors.

For all that he was still a man of his time: he was remembered long after his death in some circles less for his medical teachings than his astrological-prophetic works. Medieval necromancy and a whiff of the diabolic still hang around medicine, this being implicitly recognised by the public attention that used to be given to the supposed illegibility of doctors' handwriting, Latin abbreviations and esoteric nostrums.

In Metsys's painting Paracelsus sits with his left hand grasping in a very proprietorial manner the wooden bar at picture bottom on which the inscription is carved.

Doctard

According to that indispensable contemporary trove of hip idiom *The Urban Dictionary*, the aforementioned term—a portmanteau of "doctor" and "retard"—is a medical student or doctor who wears his or her stethoscope around the neck in public in order to get noticed.

I thought all American doctors did that: certainly most of the actors who portray doctors in film and television series do it.

Number One

In *Snakes in Suits* (2007), their dig at the men who rule the world, Babiak and Hare suggest that very few people in the real world behave like the rational self-interested economic actor, for whom everything is a game of one-upmanship and winner-takes-all, irrespective of the consequences.

In fact, studies suggest that only two groups in society at large behave in a manner which conforms to this model in every experimental setting. The first group is made up of economists themselves. Exposed to a degree course in economics students actually starting behaving in the way economists say they should (see Philip Roscoe's *I Spend, Therefore I am*); this suggests that altruism and its obverse do not have a genetic basis, as some biologists claim. The second group consists of psychopaths, the most extraverted of whom seem to be able to get through life with the minimum of problems. They mimic the emotions, being themselves the most cunning masters of manipulation. Superficial charm, self-centredness, autarky and a restricted focus are their key qualities. Psychopathic behaviour is, in fact, parasitic on non-psychopathic behaviour; which must convince economic students that they have a head-start in society.

Manipulation is at the heart of modernity, as Alasdair MacIntyre keeps reminding us. And demons too, it would seem. Kevin Dutton, an Oxford academic, has estimated that for a modern society to thrive, it needs its share of psychopaths—he puts the figure at an alarming ten per cent—who then have to be encouraged to take up careers as surgeons (imperturbable under stress), venture capitalists (coolly gambling with vast sums of other people's money) or customs officials (guards of the threshold with a flair for smelling anxiety) in order to develop their signal emotional vacancy in social rather than antisocial settings.

All the gas

"It's the latest thing," he said. "What is it?" I asked, gazing at the rows of suits and T-shirts sitting around an elliptic table in the far part of a smart Singapore coffee-shop, brightly illuminated bottles displayed before them in cabinets with sunk lighting and seats in soft pastel colours.

Then I saw the nasal cannulas, and guessed as he told me: "It's an oxygen bar. They say the stuff removes toxins and boosts the immune system." "But our bodies are adapted to the exact amount of oxygen in the atmosphere," I replied, "so what they're doing is the modern equivalent of believing in phlogiston."

Suspecting that my friend himself had visited this bar a few times before in order to sniff on the rubber, I didn't tell him—this child of the ether—that his personal cloud of purity was the most dangerous, reactive, corrosive gas in the atmosphere; and that if it did anything to him it would be to make him self-combust that bit quicker. For our material lives are lived in a state of controlled burning, and the fuel is diatomic oxygen. We call this process *time*.

An asphalt Voltaire

"There was just one other thing", said the patient, even as she made to get up out of the chair and leave the consulting room.

GPs hear this phrase, or variants of it, all the time. It is a signal that the patient is about to tell you about the soul-crippling changes that are really distressing her, and which brought her to the surgery. "I know you're busy, doctor, but…"

Then I realised that for the previous ten minutes she had been sounding out whether I could be trusted with the real reason for her attendance. There are many levels of trust to be tested in our self-exposure to others. You have to trust a listener before you can burden him with the rich seams of your own embarrassment. And that will never be a person with an agenda. And listening properly means hearing whatever's being said (and not said).

Discomfited by our mutuality, suddenly realising that she was starving—starving of the opportunity to talk—I tried to put her at ease with a joke: just think of me as a cab driver who takes confessions on the side. "Except that I haven't told you where we're going", she riposted.

Back home, where else?

Now!

Ludwig Wittgenstein writes at the beginning of *Philosophical Investigations* (§ 20, 21) that it is easy to imagine "a language consisting only of orders and reports in battles.—Or a language consisting only of questions and expressions for answering yes and no. And innumerable others.—"

As an example of the categorical imperative he could have taken the commands barked out by a surgeon to the scrub nurse or assistant: "Scalpel!" "Forceps!" "Retractor!" (After all, surgery is a kind of battle, only one that takes place in a theatre.) Sometimes these curt explanations are the only sounds to be heard beneath the focussed lights and in the concentrated silence of the operating field. They mark a hierarchical command-chain (as in the army), but also make it plain that the success of surgery depends on rapid expedition. The relationship is not as asymmetrical as it sounds.

To obtain what he (or increasingly she) needs the surgeon utters a nominal imperative, in which a more intricate verbal instruction is implied: "Give me the scalpel!", "Hand me the forceps!" or "Insert the retractor!" The compression of a phrase into a single word suggests that intention, utterance and action are almost synchronous. Irony is impossible. It is as if the voice commanding St. Augustine to open the Bible as related in his *Confessions* had merely snapped "Book!"

As Wittgenstein puts it in his rather laboured way, so many assumptions about language are built into single word sentences. Nobody is going to look at the instrument in question in order to understand what such sentences *mean*. All that needs to be uttered is the name of the object whose presence is required; the word is a *summons*.

The event-collector

Now the event assumes dimensions which ordinary events never seem to have taken on before. The one referred to by professionals as "traumatic" is automatically thought to induce a kind of stupefaction that makes ordinary life thereafter impossible, offers no enlightenment, and promises to blight the life of the subject for years to come. Its pathogenesis acquires mythical proportions, and indeed is experienced as a kind of negative miracle. Chronology and causality become so enmeshed in the event that it proves impossible to disentangle them. Collectors go in pursuit of it and can talk about it from experience: it is considered presumptuous for anyone to talk about it unless he has been on the scene in person—he must have been a *witness*.

The event-collector has the authority of this deeper knowledge. He brings calamities to word, and believes nobody should prey on disasters unless he has the accreditation of being the person-who-was-there. He can tell you about events if you prompt him, because all event-collectors bask in the deep modesty of their superior knowledge; he can even reel off for you the dates of his catastrophes.

Kaposi sarcomas

I used to get the curious impression when reading some of the AIDS memoirs that appeared in the early days when the disease first emerged in France that the only medicine strong enough for a life at the total mercy of desire was the very disease that was causing so much havoc. Once the diagnosis had been made a kind of inner calm descended on the afflicted person, though the prognosis in the 1980s was so often poor.

Then I was assailed by the horrible thought that this was precisely how the market operates: an enormous hydra-headed machine that makes so many people feel inadequate, lonely, imperfect and estranged from themselves, while simultaneously offering a palliative for the emptiness and lack it has created. A fatal solace.

THE CULT OF VESTIGES

The *Journal of Pineal Research* is a reputable scientific monthly that brings together research on the organ Descartes believed on account of its anatomical localisation to be the principal seat of the soul, "and the place in which all our thoughts are formed." Although his knowledge of its anatomy and physiology was not accurate, even for his time, one of the reasons he gave for thinking that the mobile pineal or *conarion* functioned as a kind of wind-bladder for the animal spirits was that it was only structure he could find in the brain "which is not double." It must therefore be responsible for unifying the impressions which enter by so many double organs, allowing our faculties of sensation, memory and imagination to work together. "The slightest movements of the part of this gland may alter very greatly the course of these spirits, and conversely any change, however slight, in the course of the spirits may do much to change the movements of the gland." In fact, this tiny (8 mm) pine-cone-shaped structure at the base of the two hemispheres is of considerably greater importance in vertebrate mammals than humans, who, Descartes believed, were alone in possessing it: in rodents, for example, it is purely endocrine and lacks neurons. However, it does secrete melatonin—the beneficial "hormone of darkness"—and seems to have a role in delaying sexual maturation.

Because of the strong similarity between the pinealocytes and the photoreceptors cells of the eye some evolutionists believe it to be implicated in the cycle of circadian rhythms; Madame Blavatsky considered it the mystical third-eye; and Georges Bataille—not to be outdone—the black-box of Western rationality, the black-box being a systems engineering term for a node in a circuit of relations that processes information without its users having explicit knowledge of its internal workings, which thus remain "obscure".

Open Data

"The facts speak for themselves, don't they?" This is a phrase commonly heard in these neo-liberal days when those who believe in free enterprise also subscribe to the view that even though statistics may be misinterpreted, in the long run the Invisible Hand (or the free play of opinion) will filter the cacophony and ensure that truth prevails. Facts are self-evident, "evidence" being that which is apparent of itself (*ex video*). The more thoughtful subscribers to this view—which has its origins in utilitarian philosophy—will have read Francis Galton's observation that the crowd at a county fair more accurately guessed the weight of an ox when their individual guesses were averaged than either their own estimates or those of cattle experts taken in isolation.

Sceptics and anti-positivists, on the other hand, know that facts *never* speak for themselves, and can all too easily be massaged or manipulated. Data, they suggest, are dangerous without metadata. They can all too easily be manipulated. Who gathered the statistics, by what means and for what reason? They want to know how much confidence can be attributed to them. Raw data need dressing. People bring perspectives with them. Sceptics will point to rational bubbles when groups of people make very poor decisions based on what they think are the facts. Neither group is likely to make any sense if it doesn't know that Galton was actually referring to the median—the middlemost reckoning in a spread of values—and not the mean or average.

There is a much deeper problem with probability theory in medicine. It gives with one hand and takes away with the other. It invites patients to live in an *as if* world, although nobody ever lives there. The average, and other kinds of statistical odds, certainly exist, but only in a ghostly way: the average case in a collective group is an abstract, and bears only a tangential relation to the individual person. The average can have no impact on a system of which it itself is the epiphenomenon: that is the key point. It is a second-order attribution, and quite rightly regarded as such by ordinary citizens.

Doctor Subtilis

I sometimes tell French people when they inquire about my provenance that I'm "un anglais d'Ecosse" (if only to see whether they get the joke). The great philosopher-theologian John Duns Scotus (*circa* 1266–1308) was sometimes identified on the European continent as "Scoto Inglese". He was later accused of being a hairsplitting scholastic, and his birthplace in Berwickshire—which is subsumed into his name—has provided us with the word "dunce". Those who had rejected the old learning would contemptuously refer to those who had made an appeal to his authority, "Oh, you are a *Duns(man)*." Sometimes you really can be too subtle for your own good.

Neuroimages

Calling the products of computer tomography, scintigraphy, magnetic resonance and all the other kinds of imaging *scans* is hardly an anodyne act. It suggests that these images, which are in the last instance both the archival records and the artefacts of a highly technical culture, offer a direct empirical "slice" of reality—which in the most lurid of cases, with fMRI, *is* brain activity. It is to suggest that there are biochemical processes and events which, by their very nature, are the sufficient causes of human actions. Yet a "brain scan" is a composite, manipulated image of blood-oxygen levels in the cerebral microcirculation: it doesn't provide an "index" (indexical images are direct mechanical imprints like a brass rubbing or a coin of the realm that bear a direct material relation to what they show) of brain activity itself, although hundreds of articles implicitly invite us to share the supposition that it does—"as if a magic lantern threw the nerves in patterns on a screen," in T. S. Eliot's phrase. The courts are now confronted by defence lawyers who seek to shift the blame from culture to nature, as if the acts committed by their defendants bore some kind of causal relationship to their biology (in which case, of course, the very term "actor" becomes an empty one).

Although we may have the impression that technology is bringing us closer and closer to the very nature of material reality, we are in fact slipping more and more into the realm of representation. Brain scans, while denoting magnetic field changes within our physical substance, also go to work as performative signs, convincing more and more unsuspecting subjects that their subjectivity, as brought to light in this disincarnate spectre, is an *object*. These images are at most correlates of consciousness, and even that is a topic of some conjecture.

Evidence, as it has conventionally been understood, will become indeterminate, prejudicial as much as probative, and reason—as is apparent now if not to the early pioneers of the modern—a kind of magic. After all, what we have is a body reconstituted in 3D, already inside its own sarcophagus.

Pharmakon

It was the philosopher and deconstructionist Jacques Derrida who, in "Plato's Pharmacy", put us on to the rather extraordinary collision of meanings in pharmacology. Our word "dose" came into English from late Latin via French; it ultimately derives from the Greek word *dosis*, a portion prescribed or, more prosaically, something given, a term used by the Greek physicians for an amount of medicine. It is ultimately related to our words "date", "donation" and "data," which all derive from the past participle *dare*, to give or offer. A dose is something given (even "a dose of the clap").

In English, something given gratuitously is a "gift". In German and the other Germanic languages, however, "das Gift" is the standard term for "poison", a word English took over from the Romance languages. Like the Greek term *pharmakon*, it indicates that what might be a remedy can also be toxic. Apollodorus tells us in his work *Bibliotheca* that Asclepius, the Greek god of healing, had received a magic potion from Athena derived from the blood of the Gorgon: taken from her left side it destroyed the patient, taken from her right it saved. No wonder Derrida made the *pharmakon* an emblem of undecidability.

But it was the medieval physician Paracelsus who left us the classic maxim of toxicology: "Alle Dinge sind Gift, und nichts ist ohne Gift, allein die Dosis macht dass ein Ding kein Gift ist." ["All things are poison and nothing is without poison; only the dose makes a thing not a poison".] This is often and conveniently shortened to the adage: "the dose makes the poison." In other words, substances may be beneficial in low doses and harmful in high ones.

Ordinary water, that pure life-bringing substance, can become a poison if too much of it is taken in too short period of time. Andy Warhol is alleged to have died of water intoxication owing to an uncontrolled infusion after a routine gallbladder operation.

Antipsychiatry and the market

Adam Curtis, in his documentary series *The Trap*, makes an important connection between the anti-psychiatric ideas of R.D. Laing, in which family interactions were modelled on notions of game theory cribbed from Gregory Bateson, and subsequent developments in therapeutics. Laing's disbelief in the reality of psychiatric labels was assimilated to a deep pop-cultural suspicion about the "state" as an insidious organiser of the personal life. In one notorious experiment psychiatrists sympathetic to Laing's counterculture notions presented themselves, in a frankly deceptive manner and without much of a methodology, as mentally unstable at a number of institutions in the US and were admitted as patients (the Rosenhan experiment).

This event had two major fallouts: trust in the expertise of psychiatrists to diagnose (and therefore treat) mental illness was shaken to the core, and the companies manufacturing medications for psychiatric disorders altered their strategies. Now they advocated a behaviourist strategy based on checklists and the externalisation of psychological symptoms thought to be indicative of anxiety and depression. The American Psychiatric Association revised its diagnostic practices and shifted the profession to a more reductionist model of mental illness. Patients would have to be taught to exhibit the appropriate symptoms and in general behave more predictably, like machines. This might sound like a form of conspiracy theory, but in many respects it followed a logic dictated by the market, which encouraged self-diagnosis of effects (symptoms) rather than causes. It became possible to go on a long course of an antidepressant simply by meeting a set of diagnostic criteria; the prescribing physician didn't have to know anything about the patient's previous life. A sense of the complexity of the individual patient was banished, since talking slowed down throughput and hindered "efficiency."

What the 1980s witnessed, first in the US and then everywhere else, was an unwitting collusion of arguments from both sides of the political divide: hospitals for the mentally ill were closed because the Left believed institutionalisation in any form was wrong, and the Right because they cost way too much money. The decade also witnessed Michel Foucault, darling of the radical Left, write several articles late in his life in favour of economic liberalism: he thought it would be a "much less bureaucratic... and disciplinarian" form of politics than the welfare states that had emerged after the Second World War

Emotion Studies

It is surely the case that the contemporary investment (in all senses) in neurobiology with the grotesquely sinister implication of an enforceable empathy is an attempt to extend rationalism on the assumption that the emotions (can be made to) work on causal principles too. In a material world subject to the physical laws of the universe, why shouldn't the emotions follow the same kind of manipulative logic? Wanting to read the emotions cognitively rather than collaboratively is in fact how an autist proceeds.

If emotions were produced according to a causal principle, then they would indeed be conditional and controlling. But they don't work like that. Emotions are elaborate kinds of disclosures and beckonings, signs that reveal us to ourselves. They are ethical ways of apprehending the world, and yet we are largely clueless about them. Nothing is more intimate, and yet our emotions often deceive us. And as David Hume recognised in his *Treatise* without them reason has no steadying ground. For the bothersome thing (though it didn't greatly bother Hume) is that we cannot determine what we should do in our short time in this world from any fact about it.

More body parts

Why do we utter "My foot!" as a dismissive ejaculation? "Is it because it is even lower by one measure than the arse, which stands halfway between foot and head but still is understood to be the bottom—or 'bum'—and therefore spiritually lower than the foot? And thus the foot, because physically the lowest, is able to work as a euphemism for the lowly arse, which I, in a gesture of politeness, substitute prissily for ass, opting for the English form as against the American", writes William Ian Miller in *Faking it*. (I hate to disillusion the intrepid Professor Miller, who is a true stylist among academics, but plenty of British people are quite happy to interject "My arse!" loudly into conversation.)

The French interject a sarcastic "mon oeil!" in similar circumstances. We need to be wary of physiological essentialism, where the lower parts of the body are automatically accorded lower status too. In French the foot has a much more positive association than in English: "C'est le pied!" mean "It's great!" where referring to the foot means you got a kick out of whatever it was you were doing. This same, lowly part of the anatomy can even be used by lovers, as in the question: "Tu prends ton pied?" To "have your foot" means to reach an orgasm. It comes directly from the Latin phrase "pedem tollere", one of Cicero's little jokes. There is no direct English equivalent, but it could be said to be the consequence of the expression "spread a leg".

Sign language with accents

Reading French psychoanalysts leaves you with the distinct impression that psychoanalysis isn't so much about finding new therapeutic possibilities for the suffering individual in bourgeois society (although it has been a useful source of revenue for professional woe-warmers) as to provide a new kind of semiotics for intellectuals—one in which omniscience can luxuriate in the spectacle of its struggle with willing and believing.

"J'ai mal"

In his book *Medical Nemesis*, which is now well over half a century old, Ivan Illich points out that, in French (and other Romance languages), bodily pain is synonymous with evil. This subtle charge escapes the Germanic languages which have many other synonyms for the harrowing experience of being alone with one's own bad news, but nothing that quite surrenders existential and social being to the clutches of Beelzebub in the same way as the French does. In my experience *douleur* (the word we would translate as "pain") is used almost exclusively by the French to indicate point-specific pain—cardiac, tonsillar, lumbar—while *mal* is used for more nebulous, ontological, difficult-to-define states of not feeling quite right. (The best known of these would be *mal de foie*, which has often been advanced to me by French patients as an explanation for their not feeling well on those occasions when I've been at a complete loss to tell them why.)

In his famous *Essays on Theodicy*, Leibniz distinguishes between three kinds of "malum". "Evil may be taken metaphysically, physically and morally. *Metaphysical evil* consists in mere imperfection, *physical evil* in suffering, and *moral evil* in sin." And even though we may have as little time for Leibniz's metaphysics as we have for alchemy, it is nevertheless true that our imaginations are still under the impress of concepts that originated in metaphysics. That is why some philosophers talk of "algodicy": the attempt to explain the nature of suffering in a world where God is dead and there is no ultimate meaning. But of course our lives have meaning. So how can we bear the pain?

At which point we realise we have become political beings of a rather special kind. Gone is the sympathy which Adam Smith thought would regulate the world if we all acted in our own best interests; in comes the cold, emotionless observer who is determined to be nobody's fool. At the best it is the attitude of a natural scientist or a stoic humanist (Miroslav Holub); at the worst it affects a cynically hard affirmation of evil.

A PERFECT PROFESSION

The one thing people know about the Greek philosopher Empedocles, thanks to the dramatisations of Friedrich Hölderlin and Matthew Arnold, was that he stepped into the active crater of Etna in order to demonstrate his doctrine of re-incarnation to his disciples and prove to them that he had become a god. A single man wanted to go up in a blaze and become a universal principle.

Probably the last philosopher to write in verse, Empedocles was famed in his lifetime for his brilliant oratory, knowledge of natural processes including the organs of the body and "drugs that exist for ills and old age", and his talents as a public health physician—in warding off epidemics. This he seems to have done by improving the water supply and burning infected articles: a historically attested plague at Selinus was halted by the practical applications of the philosopher's observations. Because of his ability to catch by means of animal skin bags the hot desert winds that perished the crops on Sicily he was known as the Windstopper. Although this is a magic trick mentioned in the story of Aeolus in the Odyssey, Empedocles may simply have had a series of windbreaks erected. At any rate, he was convinced that he merited his Delphic wreath and was an "iatromantis"—a physician-seer in the manner of Apollo and Asclepius. Humans, Empedocles taught, are actually higher beings who for some unspecified crime have been condemned to eke out a miserable existence on earth. Cycle after cycle goes by until, through observance of the proper virtues, they finally get to exist in one of the higher forms: as prophet, doctor and poet. From there, it is only a change of sandals to godliness.

This might be compared with Socrates' lyrical words on the pteronymic strivings of the soul to behold true being; if it falls back to earth then the law ordains that the soul that has seen most of truth will be placed "in the seed from which will be born a philosopher": doctors only come in fourth place along with athletes, behind righteous rulers (second) and businessmen (third), but ahead of prophets (fifth) and poets (sixth).

The only hope

We are living, at least in the West, in the days of the health religion. And whoever doubts it is a blasphemer.

Claudio's famous lines for the down-at-heart in Act III of Shakespeare's *Measure for Measure*—"The miserable have no other medicine but only hope"—have been reversed.

Now the miserable have no other hope but only medicine.

Measure this

In Georg Büchner's play *Woyzeck*, the unfortunate main character has to live on a diet of peas in order to provide the Doctor with scientific data: he is a laboratory specimen, whose reactions are subject to regular checks. His emotions are measured too. At the devastating moment when the Officer suggests to him that his wife Marie is being unfaithful, the Doctor examines him with evident pleasure. "Give me your pulse, Woyzeck your pulse!" he tells him. "Brief, violent, skipping, erratic... Facial muscles tense, occasional spasms. Bearing agitated, tense."

Woyzeck's suffering has been just indexed as an array of physiological responses. In Büchner's astonishing fragment of a play, *Woyzeck*, based on an actual murder in Leipzig in 1821, the uneducated, mentally fragile man at the bottom of the social order is the character who thinks; and because he thinks, feels pain. The real victim however is his wife Marie, whom he kills.

What fascinated Büchner about Woyzeck's suffering? The German culture critic Theodor Adorno wrote in his book *Aesthetic Theory* that "rational cognition has one critical limit which is its inability to cope with suffering" and Arthur Kleinman, in his influential *The Illness Narratives*, regretted that clinical and behavioural science had "no routine way of recording this most thickly human dimension... of illness." That didn't stop the development of psychometric visual analogue scales in the later part of the twentieth century. A patient told me about having a ruler marked 0 to 10 thrust into her hand without a word of explanation by a nurse in the obstetric ward of one of Strasbourg's main hospitals when she was admitted in early labour. What could be more threatening to a professional than to have to acknowledge fellowship with a suffering human being, especially one as vulnerable as a parturient woman?

Symptom scales, survey questionnaires and checklists, as a psychoanalyst friend once said, are "blatantly obvious devices for keeping patients at bay."

Word-beasts

Galen commonly compared his patients' characteristics to animals—such and such is a dog, or a snake. He even depicted fever—a paroxysmal disease in its own right and not merely a symptom for physicians in the Roman world—as an animal whose movements had to be tracked and outwitted. He had no compunction about vivisecting real animals, which he did at public events: the primary purpose of these events was to demonstrate his anatomical prowess in competition against other physicians. He dissected cats, pigs, monkeys, baboons, dogs, snakes, fish, birds and even an elephant. One of his specialties was to open the thorax without rupturing the delicate pleural and pericardial membranes, and then locate the muscles and fine nerves responsible for breathing and the vocal cords: the beast would howl, but this was part of the show; and to the audience's marvelment he could silence and revive its screaming by tightening or loosing a ligature around what is now called the recurrent laryngeal nerve.

When dissecting the brain of a live animal he preferred to use a pig or goat since he writes (in *On Anatomical Procedures*) that the expression on the face of a monkey being vivisected disturbed him. Susan Mattern in her biography *The Prince of Physicians* observes that this aside "is a rare comment on the ethics of vivisection"—although it has to be said that the acknowledged suffering is all on Galen's side. The monkey's expression made him lose his habitual imperturbability.

PARTIALITIES

In a famous article the Harvard psychiatrist Leon Eisenberg made a distinction between *brainlessness* and *mindlessness* in psychiatry. What he didn't say was that he was giving new life to an old idea from early nineteenth-century German alienism: those doctors called *Psychiker* attributed mental diseases to emotional conditions while *Somatiker* saw them as being due to physical causes and brain disorders. With Greisinger's contention that "mental diseases are brain diseases", the *Somatiker* won out for most of the century, giving rise, in the rational nosology of Kraepelin, to the modern system of psychiatric categories.

Most of the twentieth century, in the wake of Freud and psychotherapeutics, was marked by a partiality for psychodynamics and the social-personal aspects of mental illness—psychiatry therefore "brainlessly" neglected how cerebral processes might intervene.

Going into the twenty-first century it is all too obvious that we have embraced the opposite, crassly reductive trend of extreme biologism or "mindlessness." This is what you get when you adopt the Cartesian position on the mind-body but refuse to incur its somewhat inconvenient metaphysical baggage—it is only by having dualism in the background that materialism can disregard "mind" and interpret behaviour in terms of plain brain matter.

Neither approach can of course do justice to the sheer complexity of mental illness and to the demands of patients. It might even be suspected that such reductivism is a response to the sense of fright and fear which mental illnesses arouse in us, even among carers. Just as human illness needs to take account of emerging zoonotic diseases and their relationship with the environment (and environmental policies), mental illness needs to consider psychological, biological, personal, familial and social aspects of the person. Living things are creatures of need.

All of which takes time, and there's no money in it.

THE BENEFITS OF THE NEGATIVE

"Humanity is overrated," quips Dr Greg House, in one of the most popular doctor series on the box. It's not so much the grand issues of life and death which carry this series, though they're hardly absent, but the cane-wielding Dr House (played by Hugh Laurie), who manages to get away with being both a rather British type of misanthrope and junkie (his drug of choice is Vicodin®, a semi-synthetic morphine derivative) by virtue of his ability to solve diagnostic dilemmas that would have stumped the combined efforts of Dr Watson and Sherlock Holmes. House's scriptwriters have patently ignored the advice of Dr. Cox in Samuel Shem's novel *The House of God*: "Newbie, do you happen to know what a zebra is? It's a diagnosis of a ridiculously obscure disease when it's much more likely that the patient has a common illness presenting with uncommon symptoms. In other words, if you hear hoof-beats, you just go ahead and think horsies—not zebras." In *House*, everybody thinks zebras all the time. That's because it's a detective series masquerading as a medical one.

Like the philosopher Friedrich Nietzsche, House is convinced that showing pity means losing vital energy. He tells his colleague Cameron forthrightly that her emotions are clouding her judgement. And he has no time for the pieties of patient autonomy: the good patient is the one who surrenders without let to the glare of his clinical acumen. Indeed, the drama's screenwriters have cleverly recognised that by bestowing more than the usual quota of negativity and radicality on House, they can make his character even more persuasive: his abrasive, odiously intelligent, often overbearing personality is generally accepted by the sick as a *benefit*. The crisis point then becomes a moment of revelation. The "unity of opposites" is seen from a new standpoint. And the viewer becomes the addict.

Another quip from House: "Patients sometimes get better. You have no idea why, but unless you give a reason they won't pay you." The writers of the series are evidently well-read, since we find Heraclitus expressing a similar sentiment about the role of money in medicine: "Having cut, burned and poisoned the sick, the doctor then submits his bill." The issue of being paid for services to humanity is likely to remain an unresolved one, however: to the despair of the administrators in the one hospital that is prepared to employ him, House regularly fails to submit his bills.

Heraclitus's saying has another meaning, one even more applicable to the House phenomenon. The philosopher was referring to the terrifying pre-anaesthetic medical practice of *temnein kai kaiein*—cutting and cauterising. Harm and hurts—evils to be avoided in the healthy state—would be deliberately applied by doctors, and accepted by patients, for the sake of ultimate remission. A great disturbance in the universe becomes a force for good. Jung would have recognised House as a type of the wounded healer.

But when have we ever seen a doctor treat his patients as an inconvenience, if not a downright waste of time, regarding them with the eye of Sun Tzu in his 2500-year-old treatise *The Art of War*? (House, by the way, can hold his own in Mandarin, as well as in Hindi and Spanish.) "The ill person is the tactical, the illness the strategic object of medicine." It was in fact the German soldier and writer Ernst Jünger (1895-1998) who wrote that aphorism— but it is the kind of thought that Dr House, were he less busy visiting X-rated websites, might have scribbled on the back of a prescription pad.

Institutionalising altruism

Kenneth Minogue comments wryly on the kind of internationalism that flourished after the defeat of the Nazis—that "no question arose of a monastic or ascetic idealism being required of those who worked for the betterment of mankind." All too true: the World Health Organization was lavishly resourced in the beginning, and since its universality was subject to the principle of equal distribution of posts among member states it became a matter of prestige for the leading doctors of the most obscure countries to secure an appointment at the global institute for the administration of pity. But ever since its foundation, the resources have dwindled and dwindled: philanthropy has never been more talked about, and never seemed so conceptually empty.

Are you hot?

Nowadays we practise the medicine of satisfying desires. The market creates the demand for medical enhancement just as it supplies the technologies to satisfy that demand. Such is the peculiar and perverse genius of consumer capitalism: it is able to seed alienated and self-spectating lives (starting with *Madame Bovary*) among the members of previously intact communities while offering a solution or treatment that seems to remedy to the very disorder it is busily creating. The market is even now at work producing thousands of individuals who feel unhappy with their lives and loves, their personal appearance, even the way they feel at the end of the day.

And rather than ask why the shape of things is circular rather than a journey where the walker can rest with a sense of well-earned fatigue at the end of the day and gather his thoughts for the next, they will come to those who practise medicine, and ask for a little pill of hope, belief and meaning.

Red eye syndrome

It was believed in Plato's time (see *Phaedrus*) that ophthalmic disorders and eye infections, including blindness, could be transmitted by visual contact alone.

In the dark

Virtue as expressed by compassion, benevolence and sympathy was always more important, as Gertrude Himmelfarb has shown, in Britain's Enlightenment than in France's: the liking for "enlightened despotism" among the *philosophes* was predicated on their disdain for the *canaille* (injudicious use of which word—*riff-raff* or *scum*—got Nicolas Sarkozy into trouble a few years ago), whereas the British, though frightened at times by their own mobs, as is evident from Hogarth's riotous engravings, genuinely believed in a common fund of moral and social obligations.

The odd thing is nobody knew what "Enlightenment" was in Britain until 1910, when the word entered the English language.

The neoplatonic doctor

Working overtly for your health, and secretly for his own salvation—Maimonides thought that the practice of medicine was one way of pursuing perfection through the intellectual love of God.

He was perhaps recalling somebody like Eustochius of Alexandria, a doctor who, as Porphyry mentions in his *Life of Plotinus*, "came to know Plotinus towards the end of his life, and attended him until his death: Eustochius consecrated himself exclusively to Plotinus' system and became a veritable philosopher." How a doctor was able to become a Plotinian with its mysticism and general contempt for the body is difficult to conceive. As the great French scholar Pierre Hadot relates, after having gone into seclusion for a month to write his famous text *Plotin ou la simplicité du regard* (*Plotinus or The Simplicity of Vision*), a sense of remove and unreality seized him when he emerged from his Paris hiding-hole to buy a loaf at the local boulangerie: "seeing all the ordinary people milling around me in the bakery... I had the impression of having lived a month in another world, completely alien to ours, and worse still—totally unreal and even unlivable."

A BALM IN GILEAD

Paris is still full of hysterical Galenists, except that the humours are now the exclusive reserve of psychotherapists, for whom the body is more than ever a hulking appendage of the incorporated mind. Unlike the ancient Galenists however, they wouldn't know how to prepare you soothing elixirs of tamarind, plum liquor and jujube or Keats's "lucent syrops, tinct with cinnamon". They won't even know how to give of themselves, for you—the analysand—are the person who has to come clean, dorsicumbent on the divan.

So if you wish to excogitate in an atmosphere of galbanum, iris, cedar, neroli, angelica and vetiver visit instead one of the fashion temples on the Avenue Montaigne or Champs-Elysées and buy yourself a tiny, exquisitely enamelled bottle of attar— "Give me an ounce of civet, good apothecary, to sweeten my imagination." Either way the bill will be about the same.

THE GREAT PARADOX

In the methodical and practical working out of its applications the natural sciences are consensual, but not their philosophy. They are, after all, committed to regarding the world in the absence of consciousness. Where is the temporal depth in matter?

And although reputedly secular, our era can barely tolerate anything that smacks of dissent or heresy.

Cut throats

In one of the gripping excerpts in his autobiography *L'âge d'homme* (translated into English by Richard Howard as *Manhood*, and magnificently subtitled *A Journey from Childhood into the Fierce Order of Virility*) the French writer Michel Leiris talks about the experience of having his tonsils removed at the age of five or six. It remained his most painful childhood memory, and it cast a doubt on the probity of his parents "who had indulged me only so as to be able to mount the most barbaric assault on my person."

Believing, he writes, that they were off on a trip to the circus, he found himself instead caged up with the old family doctor who took him on his lap and told him they were going to "faire le ménage"—"clean up the kitchen." Facing them was a white-gowned surgeon. "All I remember is the sudden lunge of the surgeon, who rammed some sort of sharp instrument into my throat, the pain that I felt, and the scream—like that of a slaughtered animal—that I let out." What had been thrust into his throat was a tonsillotome, an instrument designed to snare and guillotine the tonsils in one swift turn of the surgeon's wrist.

Undergoing this seemingly minor procedure (though tonsillectomy could—and can still—be fatal) without the merest whiff of anaesthetic was the end of childish innocence, and the beginning of the suspicion that everything pleasant was only a "beguilement" which disguised something altogether horrific and bloody, like the clots he spat out with the strawberry sherbet which his mother had him swallow afterwards. The resemblance between this scene of deception and the Orphic myth that tells of the slaughter of the defenceless infant god Zagreus, distracted by Titans bearing toys and a mirror, would hardly have escaped the author. For years afterwards, Leiris was terrified of losing his voice.

Arthur Koestler, growing up in a middle-class family in Budapest at roughly the same time, describes a similar experience of tonsillectomy in his autobiography *Arrow in the Blue*.

In his case, it was the family dentist who acted as ear, nose and throat surgeon, and the young Koestler had to undergo the fright and indignity of being strapped down to the operating table prior to surgery. His experience of "having his throat cut" also left an aftertaste: he thought he had been handed over to a malign power: he was filled with "cosmic terror" as though he had "fallen through a manhole, into a dark underground world of archaic brutality." The memory of this primal experience returned forcefully when he was arrested by Franco's forces in Malaga in 1937 and thrown into prison, a period during which he lived daily with the possibility of his own execution. He came to see it as lying behind his lifelong need to chronicle cruelty and oppression.

Koestler coined a word for this slaughterhouse assault on the person. It is a contraction of the words "archaic horror"—*Ahor*.

More than health

Health isn't enough. Now we have wellness, and its promotional promise of radiance and effulgence: wellness is the *look* of health.

Hoc est corpus

After dinner, our friend R., a former *chef de clinique,* passed on the story of the patient who was admitted under his care in the terminal phase of heart failure. Every morning, her family would bring her a fresh baguette, the tip of which she tore off and ate slowly and with delectation, in spite of her shortness of breath. Every day, the same ritual was repeated until she slipped into a coma and died, a week or so later.

Talking to the relatives after her death, R. asked them why they had brought her a fresh baguette every morning. She was a child of the last war, they explained, and being mother of a family of modest means exposed to hardship especially in the severe winters after the war, had always felt under obligation to eat for breakfast any stale bread left over from the previous day. So she had told her children that her last wish was to enjoy the taste of a freshly baked baguette. This was luxury for her.

I was so moved by his story, I forgot to ask R. if his patient was pious: I suppose she would have been. Her last wish was a simple one, but there is something charnel about it, if such an adjective can be used to describe what was clearly a kind of sacrament. Did she understand nibbling on the fresh baguette in a metonymic way, communing with the past at her own Last Supper? She could have been—at the other end of a life—one of the *effarés* in Rimbaud's poem: the five stray waifs who timidly and longingly watch the local boulanger making "le lourd pain blond." The muscular baker is another of Rimbaud's legendary workers, like the gargantuan blacksmith in "Le Forgeron"; day after day, the baker gets up before dawn to prepare the first batch of loaves. He has all the potency of a father-figure, but also embodies maternal qualities: both are there in the generative image of the soft and unrisen primary material taking on form in the oven. "De voir des blés, des blés, des épis pleins de grain, / De penser que cela prépare bien du pain?" writes Rimbaud in "Le Forgeron", about the endless ears of wheat and the promise of bread.

The oven: fiery symbol of the womb and the tomb, where the first alchemical substance was delicately placed in its blast of heat in order to allow it to rise and transform into an inner clot of dough and bronzed outer crust. The amassed force of the first sun plumped up by the second so that it, like a bodily host, can be consumed. The oven itself a kind of mouth from which food is taken. Guido Ceronetti writes "we are condemned to eat bread, we heirs of Egypt, children and slaves of the oven." Osip Mandelstam: "The word is flesh and bread. It shares the fate of flesh and bread: suffering." Ernst Jünger: "An era so well informed about Energetics has lost the notion of the enormous forces hidden in an offering of a piece of bread." (*Strahlungen*, Feb. 1945)

R. had been touched by this story (which I've heard him tell at other dinner parties) because it is so essentially a religious one: the dying woman had returned to her own childish dream of communion by allowing the still yeasty bread to leave some of its warmth in her own body, which she knew would soon be cold.

She was one of those people, R. said, who had enough kindness to help other people find life worth living. Did he mean the other members of her family or himself? I didn't need to ask.

INFINITESIMAL DOUBT

Was the study of anatomy really an *emancipation*? Now we know all about our bodies, but are cosmically forgetful. Especially about the prospect towards which the medicalisation of our bodies is moving us: *excarnation*.

A MARGINAL NOTE

"An artist is by nature a doctor, a healer. But if he does not cure anybody, who needs him?" (With or without the comma, the question is still an indictment.)

It was a phrase written in the margins of his notebook by the Russian poet Osip Mandelstam, rediscovering his lyric gifts as he wandered around Armenia in 1930 on an official mission to document the results of the latest Soviet Five Year Plan. His friend Boris Pasternak took the thought and wrote an entire novel out of it: *Doctor Zhivago*.

PERFECTION AS A PROBLEM

Are we as secularised as we believe? It was Christianity which first universalised the concept of illness, in the doctrine of Original Sin, for centuries one of the notions that shored up European civilisation. It could be that having internalised the doctrines of Puritanism so completely that we no longer recognise ourselves as being religious at all, one deep source of the contemporary dissatisfaction with medicine is its inability to reform our unregenerate nature—what Bunyan called "original and inward pollution." This was never the business of a physician, even if Christ was seen sometimes in this *hakim* guise. How odd it is then that doctors should be thought to have the answer to what are essentially religious questions when we recall that Original Sin was predicated on the *loathsomeness* of the body and its appetites!

The new asceticism

Descartes is not usually thought of as being the father of anatomy; epistemologically he most certainly was. While Vesalius and others risked their own lives cutting into the stinking empirical reality of the human body, Descartes laid the philosophical foundations of what he saw as solid knowledge—the fact that the human subject can take itself as its own object. This involved *withdrawing* from the body's empirical reality. The Cartesian body has more to do with geometry than solid matter.

Rationalism is not just a scientific method. It is also a hygienic procedure to prevent our minds from being overwhelmed by the empirical stockpiles of the Creation as rewritten by Francis Bacon. In other words, a way to disburden ourselves of our corporeal wealth. "The Lungs, the Heart, the Liver, shrunk away far distant from Man", writes William Blake in *Jerusalem*.

Metonymies

Medical cynicism has never been clearer about itself than in the writings of the philosopher Bernard de Mandeville (known as "Man devil" to his detractors), who was born in Rotterdam in 1670 and studied medicine at Leyden but spent most of his adult life in London, setting up as a physician after the Glorious Revolution and dying there in 1733. He wrote many pamphlets in support of the Whig party, including his most famous work *The Fable of the Bees*, a series of "remarks" on his earlier poem "The Grumbling Hive", in which he suggested that vices such as pride, vanity and greed could have public benefits; his speculations on morality and economic theory had a notable influence on the philosophers of the Scottish Enlightenment. His shockingly novel designs for the "dextrous Management of our selves" in the new wealth-creating society of eighteenth-century London must have been written in a deliberately gross manner, perhaps, as the historian Roy Porter suggests, to shock that right-thinking "amiable" Whig philosopher, the Earl of Shaftesbury, who claimed that humans were naturally benevolent and a flourishing commercial society was compatible with self-restraint.

Mandeville, on the contrary, saw all humans as acting selfishly, especially when they claimed otherwise. Porter calls Mandeville's method "anatomical realism". It was certainly an early exploration of false consciousness and moral posturing.

Mandeville approached the new mercantile civilisation of the eighteenth century like a dissector. Under the new civilised conditions (Mandeville was originally from the Low Countries, which had been the first nation to extend itself across the globe as a purely commercial undertaking), he makes medical knowledge provide the core of a new political dietetics focussed not on the individual but on the *social* body. After all, states hardly had a good record in producing moral virtue in either their rulers or subjects. Now power and prestige were beginning to attach themselves to new aspects of society such as luxury articles and conspicuous consumption.

Like Hobbes (and later Rousseau), out of rigorously individualistic assumptions, Mandeville elaborates the binding conditions for the new collective being that people were calling, for the first time, *society*. They were its member-parts. A good society could arise from nothing other than individual self-interest if governments got out of the way and allowed this force to organise itself. Everything humans did was guided by self-interest. "Pride and Vanity have built more Hospitals than all the Virtues together", is only one of his inflammatory assertions. What kept things turning, as Mandeville saw it, was "that strong Habit of Hypocrisy, by the Help of which, we have learned from our Cradle to hide even from ourselves the vast Extent of Self-Love, and all its difference Branches".

Not surprisingly, Friedrich von Hayek was a great admirer of Mandeville's writings, seeing him not just as a moral philosopher but as a keen psychologist who adopted an empirical stance to the development of society: he even went so far as to claim that Darwin's theory of evolution was the culmination of a way of thinking about complex functioning structures that had started with Mandeville: it wasn't elites or sages who designed and planned societies but a bustling sociability that arose naturally from the peculiarity of human passions and the obstacles they encountered.

What his detractors failed to remark was that Mandeville, brought up in the Calvinist faith of the Netherlands, was echoing what the religious rigorists were saying all along: man is a *fallen* creature, depraved without the intervention of divine grace, and bound to act viciously because unredeemed. Mandeville's novelty was to urge this fallen creature not to adopt sackcloth and ashes.

LEND ME YOUR PARACHUTE!

In her marvellous book *The Spirit Catches You and You Fall Down*, which opens with a description of birthing rituals in rural Laos, Anne Fadiman says that in the Hmong language, the word for placenta means "jacket". "It is considered one's first and finest garment"; and it has to be buried in the right manner, otherwise the baby might vomit when nursed. Or worse.

This would surely be of interest to the German philosopher Peter Sloterdijk who has a chapter in his bulky *Spheres* trilogy called "Requiem for a Discarded Organ":"obstetricians know that there are always two entities which reach the outside in successful births". The bloody sponge, he points out, is etymologically related in European languages, to the pancake: Aristotle thought the placenta was a kind of dough which allowed the child to develop: the soft gradually became solid in the uterine kitchen. Even in premodern Europe, the placenta was not treated with indifference: it had "to be guarded like an omen and brought to safety like a symbolic sibling of the newborn." It could be dried into a potent medicine, and it could be eaten too—which is what animals do. In most parts of Europe it was buried (as in Laos) and often under young fruit trees. There was a patent sympathetic connection between placentas and fruit.

Perinatal disenchantment with the unappealing object which comes slithering out of the womb "afterwards" started in the late eighteenth century; by the next century the placenta was firmly established as waste (except, remarkably, for the cosmetic industry). The original birth unit was really a dyad: phenomenologically, Sloterdijk sees the solitary confinement of individuals under modernity as beginning with the newborn stripped of its mantle—in former times the placental double could roam "among the ancestors and household spirits." Modern individualism is a "placental nihilism"; you can navel-gaze as long as you like but the knot won't untie.

The Hmong believe that when you die, your soul has to retrace the path of its life geography until it reaches the burial place of its placenta jacket, and puts it on. Only then can the soul join the ancestors; otherwise it is condemned to an eternity of wandering "naked and alone."

Immanuel Kant in the arms of Mnemosyne

Knowingly or not, choice seems to have developed as the chief weapon of social control, as an ideological mantra. Multiply the possibility of choice until there are hundreds of options: combine that with the false idea that every choice is merely optional, and you have an effective tyranny that presents itself as a voyage through a glittering emporium where everything is on offer. In fact, we are condemned to a permanent dissatisfaction, and the feeling of there always being something better we could have opted for. And everyone being master of his destiny, there can be nobody else to blame if the choice made wasn't the right one. That is what every ideology seeks to do: compel people to blame themselves rather than criticise the system.

To grasp how inappropriate rational choice theory is in the health field, it suffices to think of the genuinely ill person: nobody is less likely to want to insist on his personal autonomy or exercise the power of choice. He wants to be helped by people he can trust. He puts his life in your hands without a second thought.

The other paradox is that all meaningful choices we make in our lives begin with something that is not chosen, namely our life itself.

The Makings of a Cult Author

After the death of his elder brother Georges, the fond, wealthy and overbearing mother of the Raymond Roussel (1877-1933)—unnoticed in his lifetime except for the bizarreness of his literary productions (*Impressions of Africa* and *Locus Solus* were written using a system of formal constraints based on the sliding homophonic puns of which French boasts a great variety) and extravagantly costly self-productions of his plays—insisted that her third son should, according to his biographer Mark Ford, "undergo a medical examination *every day*." Perhaps it is not altogether surprising then that when Big Mother accompanied her son on a tour of India and Ceylon in 1910, she ensured a coffin was brought along for the voyage so as not to importune the other travellers in the event of her demise. Perhaps what is difficult to understand is why she should want to distance herself in the first place from the ministrations of the medical profession. She could well have afforded to take a doctor along instead of her son.

The Winged Messenger

It is a nice historical irony that the wand of Hermes (a winged staff with two serpents entwined) was adopted as a symbol by the American medical profession in its glory days, when MD meant "more dollars": it had been confused with the rod of Asclepius, which has only one snake coiling around an axis. The caduceus is the symbol of commerce, Hermes being not only the classical gods' parcel-service man but also the honorary protector of an unlikely union of trades: merchants, shepherds, gamblers, liars and thieves. As chief psychopomp, he also led the dead to their final resting place in the subterranean realms, and so might seem to be a more appropriate emblem outside an undertaker's office than a physician's.

The *Classical Journal* comments, disingenuously it might be thought: "The long-standing and abundantly attested historical associations of the caduceus with commerce, theft, deception, and death are considered by many to be inappropriate in a symbol used by those engaged in the healing arts." In fact, the Homeric hymn to Hermes suggests a close association between the fleet-footed god of the fat purse and Apollo, who first gave the caduceus to him as a gesture of friendship: Asclepius was the "son of Apollo." In any case, the snakes themselves are of very ancient pedigree and may represent a god, being already found as an image of the Mesopotamian god of the underworld Ningishzida, a thousand years before its first appearance in Greece.

Granularity

We live in awe, perhaps even fear, of people with prodigious memories, because the integrity of our lives is predicated on our forgetting the details of our experience whereas those who remember everything seem, like Orpheus, to be not just in love with Eurydice but with the shadowy figure of death behind her. What we forget secretly nourishes us.

Perhaps because total recall seems a terrible fate, we can't help but remember the protagonist of Jorges Luis Borges' story "Funes the Memorious", the famous story about the teenage gaucho who falls from a horse and strikes his head on a stone. Thereafter he is bedbound, although he has prodigious powers of recall. He can reconstruct a whole day, though doing so would take him another; he can remember every moment in its particularity, even the weather and cloud formations on any given day. The "graininess" of his experience prevents him from generalising or abstracting, or even undertaking any kind of analytical thought, and he is constantly being startled by his own reflection or the movement of people in space. His world, as the narrator says, is "almost intolerably precise." Not just precise, but perfect. He is sealed in a kind of echo chamber of intentionality, with the memories echoing the first salvo of intentionality in relation to an event in the world with a second kind of intentionality related to the something that was once experienced, elaborated ad infinitum.

That perhaps is how we imagine an infallible memory. Pedantic and exacting, and like all granular things abrasive. But also completely sterile: the sands of memory don't get blown anywhere. It is epistemologically inexact to say that Funes is "remembering" at all, since he hasn't forgotten anything in the first place. He is, so to speak, ineradicably self-present. Which is a curse, since no rational or imaginative thought can take place without our discarding things. (The clinical instance of this phenomenon is the journalist Solomon Shereshevsky, reported by A.R. Luria in his *Mind of a Mnemonist*, whose inability to forget—he never took notes because he could recall a speech word for word—became a lifelong torment to him. Luria also hypothesised that Shereshevsky had "fivefold synaesthesia", in which stimulation of one sense produced a reaction in another. "Once I went to buy some ice cream," he wrote. But the vendor replied to him in such a disagreeable tone "that a whole pile of coals, of black cinders, came bursting out of her mouth, and I couldn't bring myself to buy any ice cream after she had answered in that way...")

Marcel Proust, on the other hand, was facing the other way. He insisted in his concept of memory on its involuntary nature and suggested that attending to the retrieval of experience upset the mechanism. It is necessary to forget in order to be struck by reality returning when we least expect it.

Man with a tin cup

Alastair Reid grew up in Whithorn, in the south-west of Scotland, where his father was a Church of Scotland minister. He used to say that his love of the itinerant life (he became Scotland's literary representative to the Hispanic world and a favourite of the old *New Yorker* magazine under the celebrated Mr Shawn), came from the "tinkers" who came over the Irish Sea to Galloway for seasonal jobs. "They always came by our house next to the church. I used to ask my father, 'Where are they going?' And he would say, 'They don't know.'" He told Jim Campbell in an interview three-quarters of a century later that he could still recall the excitement generated by this reply.

Doing a social visit as a young GP on my rounds one morning in the same part of the world, the lady of the manse mistook me for one of those very tinkers when I rang at the front door to her farm in the Rhinns. I must have been wearing my rugged Australian stockman's coat to protect me from the weather, and she hadn't spotted my Gladstone bag. When I said that I was the trainee doctor come to see her bedridden father she was profusely apologetic, although I was more amused than insulted to be identified as a tinker. But I remember once comparing Alastair Reid to the rider in Kafka's fragment "The Departure" who, when asked where he's headed, replies "Away-from-here – that is my goal."

Health and hiddenness

Health is one of those shy and ticklish words that cannot be talked about at any great length without compromising its essential nature. It is healthy reason, argues Franz Rosenzweig in *Understanding the Sick and Healthy*, not to ask what the essence of "health" might be.

Or, to argue in naturalistic terms, it is like the religious propensity, which, if it *is* an evolved trait, has been worried to death by agnostics—they have manoeuvred themselves into a position where they cannot benefit from it.

It is a word (sanity is another) that shrinks, under the dazzle of inquiry, into its modesty.

Tea and sympathy

The compensation for bad news in the United Kingdom is to be entitled to a cup of tea. Your long-suffering, newly bereaved and generally unflappable patient picks up the porcelain pot and pours you a cup of the lightly scented, reddish-brown infusion, a leaf or two floating on the milk. Then she pours one for herself; and you sit together mostly in silence, sipping the elixir.

This seems on the one hand to be a supremely civilised act, partaking of a lightly scented drink with the very mildest of mind-altering properties while uttering time-honoured and soothing remarks. On the other it suggests an imaginative cop-out: your patient's husband has just died, war has just broken out, and here we are with nothing better to do than drink a hot infusion of *Camellia senensis* leaves. Until it becomes apparent that the whole point of the ritual is to sit together with steam emerging from the pot and the cups sitting daintily in their saucers: commiseration needs a gentle cloud of levity. A cup of tea sipped in company (with or without milk) is a theatrical prop for learning how to play your part in the great drama of British life—although it is a prop that has only been around for close on four centuries. It is also a ritual thoroughly domesticated: eighteenth-century physicians worried that tea was such a powerful stimulant it might blast the guts of the weak, and trumpeted against its consumption.

A French-speaking patient from Mali told me once that in his country they have three gradations for the gunpowder tea that is drunk nationally: the strongest, unsweetened brew is called "bitter as death", the sugary next strain "pleasant as life", and the weak third strain boiled up again from the same leaves the next day with even more added sugar, "sweet as love."

Health and efficiency

Hans-Georg Gadamer, in a rather convoluted expression that like many German circumlocutions resists wholly adequate translation but develops logically and harmoniously from its root-terms, called health *ein selbstvergessenes Weggegebensein*: a giving away [of our vital substance] while being unmindful of our selves. Health is something to be enjoyed in a general state of absentmindedness that is not quite privative but not wholly positive either. (It was the old Romantic contention—as developed by Novalis—that illness was the royal road to self-consciousness, since illness roused the unreflecting mind out of its complacency about the body, and existence in the world. For the hypochondriac, being ill might even tell him not *how* he was, but *who* he was.)

Which points another reflection: what in fact does health have to do with care? Health, as Chesterton wrote, has to do with *carelessness*. Even people who take care in order to be healthy want to be healthy in order to return to this blithe carelessness. Plato's care of the soul is a different matter altogether, something which, were it a truly living tradition would, in view of its concern for justice and the good life, obviate the need for a commentary.

In *Heretics*, Chesterton, sounding oddly like Nietzsche, suggests that when a person, or for that matter an entire people grows feeble and unproductive, it starts talking about health and efficiency. When we are vigorous we talk not about the finer details of processes, which are chains of events that we submit to, and which go on largely beyond the horizon of our will and intelligence, but about activities, which are what we do and can imagine others having done. It is therefore a sign of rude good health, of the untutored exuberance of youth, to run after ideals—the Judgement Day and the New Jerusalem, Chesterton says, rather than government-sanctioned administration of the Polypill™ and determination of QALYs (quality-adjusted life-years).

Aristotle long ago observed, in his *Metaphysics*, that the meaning of health constantly shifts its freight from *safeguarding*, as in the expression "a healthy diet", to *disclosure*, as "she has a healthy complexion."

A MAP OF SMELLS

Walking from Café Batavia to the neighbouring banjir or flood canal on Jalan Sultan Agung, a tributary of the now inadequate canal system that discharges into Jakarta's river, the Ciliwung, which itself disembogues into the Java Sea in the old harbour district at Sunda Kelapa, one of the few places in the city where you can see some of the old colonial warehouses and buildings, I was suddenly assailed.

The assault was an olfactory one: it was what our Victorian ancestors would have recognised as the "mephitic stench" of an open sewer. When I finally managed to cross the road and gain the pavement alongside the canal, I could see that the canalway was a slow-moving mire of faeces, plastic bags, dead cats and rats, and every kind of detritus. The nauseous smell could not be endured for long. This must have been what the Pontine marshes smelt like, or the fetid effluvia of the Faubourg St. Marcel which so discomfited Rousseau when he first visited Paris. This is how the "world we have lost" smelt. This was the odour of every major European city in the summers of history. This was the River Fleet in London in 1710, when Jonathan Swift wrote his lines:

> Sweepings from Butchers Stalls, Dung, Guts and Blood,
> Drown'd Puppies, stinking Sprats, all drench'd in Mud,
> Dead Cats and Turnip-Tops come tumbling down the Flood.

John Keats once wrote a beautiful couplet about "the moving waters at their priest-like task/ Of pure ablution round earth's human shores", but he couldn't have won that ecological piety from his experiences in early nineteenth-century London. In those days, the greatest city in the world was a morass of human and equine faeces, the "chartered Thames" a repellent brownish-grey sludge that also supplied Londoners with their drinking water, and caused regular outbreaks of cholera (transmission of disease by soiled water had yet to be proved). Nothing happened until the Great Stink of 1858 when the House of Commons had to be decked in curtains steeped in chlorite so that the right honourable members could go about their business unmolested by "aerial miasma". Before Pasteur's new science of bacteriology, stench was disease. The system of sewers built in the 1860s by Joseph Bazalgette and the Metropolitan Board of Works, which stretched over 2000 kilometres and took seven years to build, was one of the engineering marvels of the age. Like many of London's Victorian achievements, it is still in use.

As somebody once said, civilisation is the distance humans put between themselves and their excreta.

HEALTH AND PLENITUDE

Health in its vital processes can be considered an expression or a mechanism. Georges Canquilhem points out that if we refuse to define health and disease, asserting, like Nietzsche, that they exist on the same continuum such that there is no completely normal (or perfect) state, there are two logical conclusions. Either all men are sick, a notion which is exploited by Molière and Jules Romains, in his "iatrocratic" farce *Knock*, or all men are not sick—"which is nonetheless absurd."

It looks as if arguments for the existence of perfect health recapitulate the ontological arguments for the existence of God. And therefore have to bear the blemish of their own mistakenness.

PECKING ORDER OF THE VANITIES

There are three medical men in Flaubert's *Madame Bovary*.

There is Emma Bovary's husband Charles, who is not actually a doctor at all but an "officier de santé"—a duffer at the bottom of the hierarchical scale who has a few basic notions of diagnosis and therapeutics; it is not surprising that the ambitious chemist, the "Enlightenment man" Homais, makes common cause with him, and attempts to cajole him into doing the famous club foot "repair" in order to impress the locals. It is an operation he has no training or even aptitude for, and he famously botches it—and along with it any chance he has of saving his marriage.

Dr Canivet from Rouen is a rough, uncouth fellow with some native intelligence and skill, gathered over the years of running a practice, in dealing with bodily mishaps and illnesses. But he is not a subtle man, and his intelligence is limited.

Then there is Dr Larivière who, as the critic Allan Bloom suggests, does not really fit in the novel's plot at all. His services are called upon when Emma is dying in agony from the arsenic tincture she has stolen from Homais' dispensary and drunk. He is unable to help. He is surely—with his "long merino greatcoat" and "beautiful hands"—a portrait of Flaubert's progenitor

Achille-Cléophas, who was chief surgeon of Rouen. Flaubert grew up with his brother and sister in a wing of the municipal hospital in that city, and remembered looking through an open window more than once as his father performed a post mortem: "I can still see my father looking up from his dissection and telling us to go away."

"Disdaining all academic honours, titles and decorations, hospitable and generous, like a father to the poor, practising virtue without believing in it, he might almost have passed for a saint had not his mental acuity caused him to be feared as a demon." That confession of a disabused Aristotelian is a portrait of Flaubert himself.

Health and the Market Society

Friedrich Nietzsche, in his writings about the good life, starts from the presupposition that health and sickness are states absolute only for the unreflective person, and aims to make them overlapping—to give them unity within a continuum. Lichtenberg, in one of his aphorisms, wrote: "When one is young, one hardly knows that one is alive. The feeling of health is gained only through sickness". As a hunchback, he was speaking his own case.

Behind both these fearless German thinkers is the pre-Socratic philosopher Heraclitus, who is quoted as saying: "We know health by illness, satiety by hunger, leisure by weariness." Negative experiences are necessary for enjoying vigour, a full stomach and being able to put our legs up. And although illness is not a prerequisite for health, as hunger and exertion are for their opposites, it is only through the contrast with sickness that we know health to be a desirable thing—to be sweet.

And that is why humans should not get all they want, Heraclitus says in the same maxim—the structure of desire being such that if we got it all, nothing would be desirable. (The Qur'an says something similar: "Perhaps there is something you dislike which is best for you, and perhaps there is something you like which is worst for you.")

Heraclitus was gainsaying the inscription on the propylaeum to the shrine of Leto at Delos, which told celebrants that the sweetest thing was to get what they desired. The principal aspiration of modern market society therefore turns out to be not at all modern. It is poised to destroy the great world order based upon the unity of opposites, or, as Heraclitus would have it, the kindling and quenching of cosmic fire.

One-upmanship

The deservedly most quoted phrase in Jules Romains' classic play *Knock* is the following adage: "well people are sick people who simply don't know it." Theodor Adorno in *Minima Moralia* goes one step further. He wrote: "the very people who burst with proofs of exuberant vitality could easily be taken for prepared corpses, from whom the news of their not-quite-successful decease has been withheld for reasons of population policy."

A "healthy attitude" is therefore the new, fully integrated outlook of someone able to work on after the worst has happened. Adorno and the Frankfurt School in 1947; Louis Jouvet playing the character of Knock in the 1951 film version of the best French drama of the interwar years.

The long goodbye

The correct term for our age is *valetudinarian*.

Healthy people draw on health as a means, only very decrepit people advance health as a reason.

Rule and instance

There is no biography more like one of Dostoevsky's novels—where the *Why?* question about life has no answer other than through the love of Christ—than that of George Price, the

American scientist who came to London and got in touch with Bill Hamilton, the British evolutionary biologist and father of kin selection. Price, who had trained as a chemist and had no experience in genetics or statistics, devised the formula now known as Price's covariance equation, describing the essential interestedness, or adaptedness of altruism at different levels of organisation: an action that may seem disadvantageous to an individual may allow his or her genes to persist among relatives. With "fitness" redescribed so as to include offspring and close relatives, Price had provided a working mathematical model for how altruism made sense as an essentially economic kind of philosophical egoism that understood everything in terms of self-interest.

After a religious experience in 1970, the extreme rationalist became an enthusiastic convert. He wanted to be a Christian following the model of Jesus, and devote himself to works of charity. "My name is George," he would tell vagrants. "Is there any way I can help you?" He gave everything he possessed to the needy of north London and allowed the homeless to stay in his flat. He would sleep in his office. To his distress they stole whatever possessions he had left. In December 1974, he cut his carotid with a pair of tailors' scissors. He thought he had failed as a Good Samaritan.

Limited sociability

"No man is an island," wrote John Donne. Granted, but an awful lot of human beings seem quite happy to be enclaves.

The mystery of a life

There is an astonishing sense in early Romantic writing of people noticing each other for the first time, of being wholly absorbed by another person's life—or at least seeking to write about it. John Keats, in a journal letter (February-May 1819) to his brother George, wrote "A Man's life of any worth is a continual allegory—and very few eyes can see the Mystery of life, a life like the Scriptures, figurative..."You can find similar sentiments in the writings of Robert Burns, and in Stendhal, who is convinced that "every person—were he to succeed in getting himself fully down on paper—would be exciting and amazing and also irreplaceable," as Elias Canetti put it in a capsule biography of the French writer.

However, it was William Wordsworth who gave most memorable form to this consideration in his poem about the leech gatherer he met with his sister Dorothy on the road to Carlisle. The Wordsworths were deeply impressed by the dignity, composure and measured Scotch speech of this destitute old man bent almost double. The poet, who confesses that he has lived his whole life "in pleasant thought/ as if life's business were a summer mood", is moved to reverence by the archaic figure of the leech gatherer, "not all alive nor dead": he sees him first as a dream messenger, then "like a man from some far region sent/ To give me human strength by apt admonishment." It makes him resemble the more famous figure of the Wanderer in Wordsworth's long poem *The Excursion* who cultivated his affections "on the public roads/ And the wild paths," a figure whom the poet admitted represented himself. "He could 'afford' to suffer/ With those whom he saw suffer."

It is another kind of admonishment to realise that this old man, who could no longer eke a trade because of the diminishing numbers of *Hirudo medicinalis* in the Lake District, sold the leeches that he caught to the members of the medical profession. (Dorothy recorded his words in her diary for October 3, 1800: "He said leeches were very scarce partly owing to this dry season, but many years they have been scarce... Leeches were formerly 2/6 [per] 100; they are now 30/.)

Doctors, like poets, are singularly placed to observe the indefatigable and sometimes poignant capacity of people to endure; and by observing this capacity in others are themselves helped to endure. They only have to recall Wordsworth's famous lines written a few miles above Tintern Abbey:

> ... such [feelings], perhaps,
> As may have had no trivial influence

On that best portion of a good man's life;
His little, nameless, unremembered acts
Of kindness and of love.

Bigging it up

It's odd how Americans like to think of themselves as plain-talking, pragmatic, modern people, immune to the empty discourse of the higher metaphysics. Science talk is common sense for Americans; and they indulge it even at the risk of sounding pretentious to other speakers of English, and far removed from anything resembling sense at all. Richard Lehman notes, by way of example, that what is usually called "gut feeling" in the UK is known in the US as "clinical Gestalt."

The writing cure

The term "writing cure" can be found where we might not expect to find it: in the writings of E. M. Cioran, all of whose works are disguised autobiographical notations, and who became famous for his dismissive wit, for instance: "un livre est un suicide différé" (a book is a postponed suicide). "Writing for me is a form of therapy, nothing more," he told Fernando Savater in an interview. His first books displayed his wounds, which then became bandaged in beautifully crafted phrases as he moved from a viscerally personal style to a more aphoristic one. As his biographer Ilinca Zarifopol-Johnston writes: "The bandage—writing—is the wound's only trace and the sufferer, now a master of style, is in control of his agony. His personal agony has become aestheticized to the point that one can speak of a tortured *dandyism*."

A hospital light

W. G. Sebald's protagonist in his novel *Austerlitz* remarks on the similarity between places of punishment and places of healing.

That was certainly true of the Victorian era; and when I read Sebald's lines I was instantly transported back to the central block of the Glasgow Royal Infirmary, which was inaugurated in 1914. I did some of my training there, and rarely has a building had such a directly oppressive effect on my mood. I had no difficulty whatsoever in imagining the wards of this Bastille as places of suffering, and felt my own individuality crushed beneath its solid masonry every time I climbed the stairs to attend rounds and caught the pall of Philip Larkin's "frightening smell".

Why me?

In Jean-Jacques Rousseau's world of innocent and transparent beings coddled by Mother Nature, which is still largely ours, everybody lives in such a state of perfection it seems quite inadmissible that illnesses and accidents happen at all.

This is surely one source of the indignation with which some people greet the news of life-threatening or chronic disease. Diagnosis is a kind of lèse-majesté.

We can provide causes, so many convincing ones, but not *explanations*.

News from the Asclepium

All the gods could heal, but Asclepius made it his speciality. As a consequence, while there was considerable debate in the classical world about whether dreams had any prognostic value—Aristotle was generally agnostic about the possibility of prophesy through dreams and the Epicurians were entirely dismissive of it—those that were seeded by the healing god were of special significance. In fact, healing dreams were solicited by the sick, who would visit shrines to the deity, such as those at Kos, Pergamum or the famous *asclepeion* at Epidaurus, the most famous healing centre of the classical world, believing that because such dreams related to their personal welfare they had to be god-sent, and were of a different order from ordinary dreams. Sleeping in the *enkoimeteria*, a large dormitory attached to the temple sanctuary, supplicants had first to accomplish certain prescribed tasks (abstinence from sex and certain foods) in order to be pure enough to enter the *abaton*—the forbidden place. There they would lie flat on the ground, in intimate contact with the earth, and go to sleep: the god would visit them in their sleep and either cure them or "incubate" visions of treatment and redemption as they slept.

The idea of the oneiric pilgrimage was to be just as successful in the Christian Middle Ages and the new empire of Islam; and even the Jews travelled to the western shore of the Sea of Galilee to rest their heads on the tomb of Maimonides. It is noteworthy, however, that Asclepius, in several of his aspects (not least in his cult of the snake and the notion of patients being obliged to lie in contact with the chthonic forces of the cosmogony), is allied with the "dark mantic" forces from which his sun-god father Apollo had supposedly freed humankind by overthrowing the oracle of Gaea at Delphi.

Galen, who was a sceptic about most things and refused to accept the doctrines of the various medical schools of his time until he had verified their articles for himself, believed that Asclepius had both instructed his father to educate him in medicine and cured him of a chronic abdominal ailment in his youth. The god sent him diagnoses, prognoses and sometimes therapies: there is an instruction "On Diagnosis from Dreams" which bears his name, and Book 10 of his *On the Usefulness of the Parts* even sets out geometric arguments about the optics of the eye in obedience to a dream. Asclepius was something like his personal saviour—a psychotherapist *avant la lettre*.

Its name is Legion

The new biology threatens to render the body back to us in startling ways. Already the fundamental dividing line in life lies not between plants and animals but between eukaryotes—cells with nuclei, mitochondria and plastids (in the case of plants)—

and prokaryotes, that is bacteria. Each eukaryote is an assembly of prokaryotes; our bodies, from the biological standpoint, are *chimerae*. And while at the macroscopic level, we now have the boosterism of human rights which, riding on affluence, the English language's "soft power" and conceptual world, as well as the mistaken impression that strife has left the human scene, seeks to make the pursuit of happiness not just lawful but dutiful, the microscopic level is subjecting us to a creeping reappraisal that threatens to overturn not just the idea of consciousness as a discrete entity but to besiege the very integrity of the body. Medicine considers the body a unity, and plans with military precision restore it to order. We are not moving towards the emancipation promised by the Enlightenment, but re-assembling ourselves into a new social order, the "medieval-microcosmic". For we ourselves are societies in the shapes of assemblies, organisms, corporations and not just corpuses. Perhaps that is the fulfilment of Pascal's prediction—we have become monsters and chaos to ourselves.

Indeed, the entomologist and naturalist E. O. Wilson has written that "the pattern of human population growth in the twentieth century was more bacterial than primate." The human biomass—7.7 billion individuals at the time of writing—is however small compared to that of insects, fungi and the said bacteria, not to speak of plants. So it is that humans are both biologically puny and utterly dominant in the way we have shaped the grand scheme of life on planet Earth: the Living Planet Index states that the number of wild animals in the world has halved in my lifetime.

On being a surgeon

Harvey Cushing, the famous American "father of modern neurosurgery" and eponymous describer of the corticosteroid abuse syndrome, is said to have dissuaded a student from taking up his speciality by asking him "Do you enjoy the sensation of cutting through flesh with a knife?"

Henry Marsh, the British neurosurgeon and author of the excellent book *Do No Harm*, comes clean too when writing about his chosen speciality: "I found its controlled and altruistic violence deeply appealing."

A MYSTERY DISCOUNTED

Of all people, it is the midwife Arina Prokhorovna, in Dostoevsky's *The Possessed*, who argues for the insignificance of human life as against its being created in God's image.

Ivan Shatov, a former radical socialist who has developed religious convictions (and will later be murdered for them like Ivanov, the student whose actual killing prompted Dostoevsky to write the novel), is overjoyed to be reunited with his estranged wife Mary. He is no less delighted to become a father, even though the child Mary is carrying is the offspring of the charismatic Stavrogin, one of Dostoevsky's most troubling, Byronic characters. At the birth Shatov waxes lyrical: "It's the mystery of the appearance of a new being, a great and inexplicable mystery... There were two, and suddenly there is a third, a new spirit... a new thought and a new love... so uncanny... there is nothing higher in the world." To which age-old realisation of the magic trick performed at every birth, Prokhorovna responds with the dry laugh of mockery: "What a fuss you're making... It's simply the further development of the organism, and nothing more, there is no mystery... otherwise every fly would be a mystery. And let me tell you something. Superfluous humans shouldn't get born."

Arina Prokhorovna's deflating impulse—to spite the idiotic beatitude of the fathers in the lying-in room perhaps—was the same as that of our most famous philosophical despiser of the process of generation (Schopenhauer), although many other thinking men-midwives have said the same.

A scene which outfaces Dostoevsky's midwife occurs in Chapter 3 of Dickens' *Our Mutual Friend*. A friendless petty crook is brought in on the verge of death, and the people tending to him are all kindness and consideration: every sign of life in the dying man is treated with respect. "No one has the least regard for the man," wrote Dickens. "With them all, he has been an object of avoidance, suspicion, and aversion; but the spark of life within him is curiously separate from himself now, and they have a deep interest in it, probably because it is life, and they are living, and must die." The man revives, and becomes a malicious wastrel again; and his saviours lose their interest and respect.

Usually that vital sense of life as a force is seen in infants, as Gilles Deleuze noticed in a late essay which deals with Dickens' scene: that is why Arina Prokhorovna's blunt callousness seems all the more shocking.

THE AUTISTIC SHIFT

More than a hundred years after Emil Kraepelin, the German physician who introduced into psychiatric practice a categorical approach modelled on organic diseases for classifying mental disorders in terms of the overt signs that were taken to be manifestations of underlying disease processes—some pathognomonic, others weaker and requiring confirmation by related signs—we have still not answered the question of what a mental disease *is*. Thomas Szasz famously objected that many of those categorised as being mentally unwell ought to be divided into those who have an organic brain disorder (Parkinson's or Alzheimer's) and those whose behaviour deviates from social norms, either as judged by themselves, family or clinicians. Underlying this "liberal" approach to the whole problem, which at least has the virtue of definitional clarity and consistency, is the unthinking assumption that all social intercourse is inherently something harmonious, and towards which we strive: at one fell swoop the whole basis of that Aristotelianism looks fallacious.

THEATRE

Aristotle's definition of tragic theatre as *catharsis* or *purification* underscores the connection between the ritual event—killing of a scapegoat-victim, whether king or sacrificial beast—and the communal peace or social assuagement that follows.

Deaths on stage—which is one of the things that Aristotle mentions in his definition of "pathos," along with paroxysms of pain, woundings and "all that sort of thing"—are a sham: classical theatre generally avoided bloodshed (while reserving it for altars) as if to heighten the total make-believe of the tragedy, its distance from real violence. That is the function of the chorus: to have afterthoughts and bemoan the tragedy and point the moral, its wisdom being that of the onlooker and not the person who has gone through an experience that is visceral, mysterious and terrible.

By contrast, real bloodletting, violence and death may occur by design or inadvertence in war and medicine where the word "theatre" is also used with a dim appreciation of its origins in the rituals of primitive religion: perhaps the crucial difference is that the make-believe element in war and medicine is only partial. In both cases assuagement still follows the high drama.

Against entitlements

Despite the current piety among the right-thinking, health cannot be an inalienable human right. Were it so, then life itself is continually flouting our rights, since disease, degenerative problems and death itself are unavoidable aspects of the human condition. Nor is access to care a right: it is a *benefit*, brought about by the actions of a myriad of people, very few of whom will ever be known to us. It is a very unhelpful philosophy to live in the belief that the world *owes* us something.

A nursing icon

One of the interesting aspects of Mark Bostridge's biography of Florence Nightingale is the way it places her as an explicitly Protestant reformer in a society where the work of caring, lay and religious, was still associated with the charitable work of

Catholic societies. Her Unitarian background convinced her of the importance of good works and inspired her to devote her efforts to the improvement of society. The outcry about the death rates among the soldiers placed in the barrack hospitals at Scutari in the Crimea gave Anglican sisterhoods the opportunity to enter public life without arousing the slightest suspicion about their religious affiliations or even patriotism. But some nurses went out to the Crimea as ladies and some as women, the latter being expected to undertake the heavier, more menial and unpleasant tasks, and even in some cases to wait on the lady nurses. It was a lady's prerogative to be a manager. Such were the class divisions in Victorian Britain: philanthropy was, by definition, what a lady of better class provided to her social inferiors. What was a nurse to do, when she couldn't select her patients or, even worse, the male doctor from whom she would have to take her orders turned out (in spite of the entire profession's endeavours to be taken in through the front door and not the servants' entrance) to be a social inferior? It took Florence Nightingale a decade to convince her family to allow her to accept the post of Superintendent of the Establishment for Gentlewomen during Illness in Upper Harley Street; it was the experience gained in this post that served as an opportunity for her to campaign for improved conditions in the Crimea—which met with opposition from medical officers who wanted her to attend solely to superintending nurses.

Traditionally, if a soldier had been merely wounded on the battlefield there was every chance he wound succumb to his wounds in the field hospital. In 1705, the duc du Saint-Simon wrote: "The losses in Flanders and Italy, greater in the hospitals than in the field…". Lord Byron confirmed him a century later, being bled to death by his doctor in Missolonghi in 1825: "There are many more die of the lancet than the lance". Their assertions were still true when Britain intervened alongside the French in the Crimean War in 1854, and the Scutari barracks served as the British Army Hospital. Soldiers with injuries who entered its doors were likely to go down with malaria, cholera, dysentery or typhoid; in fact, ten times more soldiers were dying there from infectious diseases than from battle wounds. Florence

Nightingale's plea in *The Times* for a solution shocked the War office into commissioning Isambard Kingdom Brunel to design the first prefabricated wooden hospital; it was designed in six days, shipped out of Southampton and assembled on site: less than five months later it was accepting its first patients. It is thought that of the 1300 soldiers who were treated there, only 50 died, a great achievement for the time.

Nightingale improved the conditions at Scutari, ensuring that the soldiers had a better diet, ventilating the wards and having clothes properly washed (which probably reduced the number of cases of typhus). The water supply was not her concern, though the general emphasis on cleanliness must have improved wound care. Like most of her generation, she believed what her nose told her: disease came from vitiated air and bad smells. Germ theory—the evidence of things truly unseen, at least with the naked eye—had yet to enter history. Like any rationalist ascetic Puritan, what she tried to control through her policies were bodies, especially her own. She mortified herself through work and wanted to have nothing to do with her legend as the lady with the lamp, which smacked of self-glorification.

In short, her sense of purity was more religious than it was scientific. It drove her to reform nursing and hospitals for the next twenty-five years of her life. But she was empiricist enough to accept the hypothesis of bacteriological contamination when it came along. And we are still Puritan enough to associate cleanliness with godliness, purity with truth, although a visibly clean, orderly and properly regulated hospital is not necessarily one free of microbes.

The considered life

How much more difficult it is to suggest that being a great physician is not the same thing as leading an exemplary life as a physician. (The difficulty is itself the measure of the distance between medicine and philosophy.)

"THE BUSY TIME"

John Keats refers to it in one of his letters and it appears to be the period between autumn 1816 and spring 1817 during which he was duty Dresser at Guy's Hospital, while preparing his now famous volume *Poems* (1817) for the press. This role required him to stay on permanent duty for one week in three, attending to the initial management of accidents and emergencies, performing minor operations and admitting patients on behalf of the qualified surgeon to whom he was attached. Gittings and others seem to think he avoided or cut down duties at the hospital in order to attend to his poetry, but I have no difficulty in believing that an onerous working routine urged him to work on his poems. Energy fuels exhilaration abets elation.

I remember when I worked as a junior house officer in paediatric surgery at the Royal Hospital for Sick Children, Glasgow, 110 hours in the week, and I still had the energy to go out with my friends in the evening. But that kind of heroic medicine has sensibly been banned by European directives on working hours.

GODS FOR ORGANS

"Preconscious hypostases" is the somewhat unwieldy term used by the psychologist Julian Jaynes in his book *The Origin of Consciousness in the Breakdown of the Bicameral Mind*, which enjoyed a certain vogue in the 1980s, for the primitive mind-words that appear in some of the earliest literature which has come down to us, primarily that of the Greeks, "the paradigm people of Western civilisation." If we go further back, we find the ancient Egyptians had animal gods (the four sons of Horus) as protectors of the individual organs. There was Imset, human-headed protector of the liver, Hapy, baboon-headed protector of the lungs, Duamutef, jackal-headed protector of the stomach and Kebhsenuf, falcon-headed protector of the intestines.

These hypostases are markers of the assumed internal causes

of actions when other (external) causes are no longer apparent. They are key terms that locate the beginnings of consciousness in the shift from what Jaynes hypothesises as a *bicameral world*, when human beings reacted in immediate, unreflecting, obedient response to the voices in their heads. The stress of making decisions—which etymologically derives from notions of cutting and killing, in a word *trenchancy*—would be accompanied by physiological concomitants such as paling of the skin (cutaneous vasoconstriction) and cramping of the guts, panting breath and a pounding heart. These physiological sensations are respectively called *thymos, phrenes* and *kradie*. "*Thumos* is the experience of stress which moves one to action: it is not Ajax who is zealous to fight but his *thumos*, nor is it Aeneas who rejoices but his thumos... a man may speak to his *thumos* and hear from it what he has to say."

One good reason for assuming that Homer could not possibly be a single person is that the hero of the second book under his name, *The Odyssey*, is almost a modern man: we go from a martial world where a man has no more self-consciousness than his helmet to a world of subjective consciousness, where Odysseus deliberates about what he is going to do, and assumes that we will understand not just his actions but his motives and wiles too.

Our problem is that we posit "post-conscious hypostases" and fail to recognise that by creating linguistic categories we are misled into thinking them congruent with the reality they seek to demarcate. We have an enormous vocabulary to express the qualities of the psychological life. Yet the danger of our hypostases is to blind us to the person who is hidden by the schema. The organs, we might say, are external linguistic gods, and no less fearsome than the old Egyptian animal ones.

Das Werkzeug

A polysemous term in eighteenth-century German, *Werkzeug* encompassed everything from tool and instrument to bodily organ and body itself; and is found in all these senses in Novalis. A proper education in those days would see to it that a young man acquired the skills and pleasures of manual craftsmanship before those of poetry. These were some of the things made by Hephaestus: Hermes' winged helmet and sandals, Aphrodite's girdle, Eros' bow and arrows, Agamemnon's staff of office, Achilles' armour, Helios' chariot and the bronze clappers sported by Heracles.

It perhaps found its apotheosis in the conception of Gaston Bachelard, genial French philosopher of science (and admirer of Novalis), that scientific instruments are themselves forms of applied rationalism—"theories materialised". Application of the *Werkzeug* enables theoretical concepts to overcome the purely abstract nature of hypotheses and give form to truths more concrete than would be the case with ordinary empiricism. Bachelard called this "phenomenotechnics", a shift from the phenomenological description of helmets, girdles, bows and clappers to a science that gives substance to its objects.

Reverse engineering

The effectiveness of medicine participates in its historicity. Every century expurgates the preceding one clinically. The frank disinterest of most doctors in the history of their profession is itself a significant event in the history of medicine.

Anaesthetic

Medicine in the eighteenth and even into the nineteenth century, for all its efforts to acquire the status of a *respectable* profession, continued to trail the trappings of the raree-show or music hall act. The ancient drama at the heart of medicine was put fairly and squarely on stage in the public dissections of the Middle Ages or much earlier in history in the agonistic events in which Galen would compete with other physicians not only at the bedside but in rhetorical and other competitions (including animal vivisection) in front of an audience that would cheer or jeer as the mood took it, swayed no doubt by loyalties, the nature of the spectacle and its outcome.

When nitrous oxide was first produced by Joseph Priestley and further investigated in 1799 by Humphry Davy and his colleagues at the Pneumatic Medical Institution in Bristol, it initially became far better known for its intoxicant effects as "laughing gas": it was a fairground attraction. What an affront to the dignity of doctors!

It is only once nitrous oxide was properly developed as an anaesthetic agent for dentistry in 1844 (to be superseded by ether and chloroform for more ambitious surgical procedures) and patients were properly anaesthetised and kept quiet, rather than inebriated and euphoric, that medicine could assume its severely modern mask of *gravitas*.

A Chinese syllogism

There is hope if we can paraphrase Lao-Tzu.

The holy man is sick. But his sickness sickens him. Therefore the holy man is not sick.

Listening to their insides

Marcel Proust, in a marvellous passage in the second volume of his *In Search of Time Past*, has the narrator and the writer Bergotte discussing contemporary medicine and health—something Proust knew quite a bit about through his own constitutional and imagined illnesses, as well as by dint of his family's high standing in the Paris medical world (father and brother). They come to this summation of the nature of doctors: "That my doctor might be a crushing bore didn't bother me; all I required of him was that his art, the laws of which were beyond me, should enable him to examine my entrails and utter an indisputable oracle on the subject of my health."

Michael Wood seizes on this observation in his book *The Road to Delphi: The Life and Afterlife of Oracles* to show how Proust cunningly conflates two ancient practices: that of haruspication (divination by inspecting the inner organs of sacrificed animals) and consulting the oracle. We can leave aside the practice of haruspication, which historically appeared after the oracles went silent, although Proust makes much sport of the hypochondriac fantasies of people who think they can hear what their insides are saying to them. Wood devotes a whole chapter of his book to developing the parallel between medical consultation and the ancient practice of going to consult the oracle.

Sometimes the consultation of an oracle barely seems to be a religious practice at all, although a god is always rumoured to be somewhere behind the scenes—"but the oracle is certainly the most secular, and most easily secularised of religious practices." Conversely, writes Wood, "a whiff of religion" creeps into secular practices that resemble, even a little, the consultation of an oracle. For him, it is not psychoanalysis that creates the conditions for this experience, psychoanalysis being premised on a special kind of inwardness, but the simple medical consultation. Doctors give us messages and signs, oracles and omens; and increasingly the signs are not merely indicative, but productive: they rely on statistical not celestial measurements.

Heraclitus is reported by Plutarch to have written in one of his sayings, "the lord whose oracle is in Delphi neither discloses nor hides his thoughts, but gives signs." (*De Pythiae Oraculis*). Advice is always provided in indirect form, through imagery, riddle or wordplay, and although the words of the oracle were immediately understood, as the centuries passed they required interpretation. It is not a bad description of the difficulties of understanding Heraclitus' own gnomic style. As Kahn says in his commentary on the philosopher: "this parallel between Heraclitus' style and the obscurity of the nature of things... is not arbitrary: to speak plainly about such a subject would be to falsify it in the telling... The only hope of 'getting through' to the audience is to puzzle and provoke them into reflection. Hence the only appropriate mode of explanation is allusive and indirect: Heraclitus is consciously and unavoidably 'obscure'." For there may be a dread and hidden meaning to the oracles, as Oedipus discovered in adult life when he omitted to ask which man might be his father. Oracles don't mean: "they play a verbal card" as Wood writes.

It could be that what we're all looking for—and not just at the doctor's—is *authorisation*. Actions must have something more than a cause; they need a reason; and although a reason is never simply a cause, finding a reason implies uncovering a cause.

Mere appearances

Perhaps a medical training is the better way to become a phenomenologist, if Heidegger is to be taken at his word. "[In speaking of the symptoms of a disease] one has in mind certain occurrences in the body which show themselves and which, in showing themselves as thus showing themselves, 'indicate' something which does *not* show itself." In view of the fact, says Heidegger, that the term "appearance" can signify a heraldic sign announcing what cannot show itself as well as the genuine phenomenon, the "showing-itself", a certain amount of confusion seems inevitable. A clinician is trained to distinguish the phenomenon from semblance without knowing that he is palpating and auscultating *Dasein* itself.

Parenting the Buddha

At the age of 29, say the legends, Prince Siddhartha left the protection of his father's palace—in fact, three palaces—which had been expressly constructed in order to shield him from all knowledge of human distress and went among his subjects. It was the profoundly unsettling experience of witnessing suffering (*dukkha*) in the form of diseased and dying persons—in spite of his father's best efforts to remove the sick, aged and suffering from public view—which led him to meditate under the Bodhi tree for forty-nine days and then to adopt his life of asceticism, and ultimate enlightenment as Buddha. What antidote could right living bring to the perishability of the flesh? Self-immolation of the spirit insofar as it is a calculative entity, never accepting a thing for what it is. Thus the ego is fingered as the source of its own problems, much as Jean-Jacques Rousseau decided when he wrote his pedagogical novel *Emile*, which in seeking to provide an environment in which a person might retain what Rousseau believed was innate human goodness invented the life-stage we now call *childhood*.

A CHILDREN'S SONG

Robert Burns, in one of his most famous erotic poems, has "a body comin' thro the rye." A body—that is, a person. The world might not be alive, as in the animist religions, in which being was intelligible only in terms of living; the striking (female) figures moving through the landscape certainly are. We can assume that Burns, and late eighteenth-century Scottish linguistic usage in general, was still perfectly acquainted with Thomas Aquinas' theory of Being which held that there was no such object in the world as a dead body, solely the remains of a living one. It is this body which is resurrected in Christian belief, the soul being its "form". The body is alive—living, feeling, striving. It can make something of the forces that made it, and be intimate with other bodies. It was perhaps such a thought which led the later Wittgenstein to say the body is the best image we have of the human soul.

We are all thoroughgoing Cartesians now, it would seem, because the automatic association with the word "body" is the dead one: it is a corpse, a cadaver, a substrat of what was once living. Only then it is fully intelligible, another aspect of the indifferent matter that provides the tenets for our understanding of the world. As Terry Eagleton once wrote: "To announce the presence of a body in the library is by no means to allude to an industrious reader." Life—a body—is now accounted for in terms of bare matter. And such is the ontological dominance of death in modernity that Nietzsche could toss off a remark about life being merely "a special form of being dead."

Unreliable narrators

The novelist Patrick McGrath, whose father was superintendent of Broadmoor Prison, the high-security psychiatric hospital in Berkshire, likes to use doctors as narrators because they provide an almost unquestionable veneer of reliability and authenticity—until it sinks in on the reader that their motives are just as undisclosed, fly-by-night and threadbare as those of *any* narrator.

The nocebo effect

I read the poems in the Bloodaxe anthology *The Poetry Cure* (2005) and they made me feel queasy and even slightly sick. Some of them were clearly afflicted by a frightfully *gregarious* malady.

A fig-leaf

How long does Hans Castorp stay on the magic mountain? Seven years. And how much sexual congress does he experience? One hour of passion with Clavdia Chauchat on Carnival night. "Wicked [and] riotously sweet" it might have been but the sexual act itself was over in no time, which as often as not is true, in other circumstances, for intimate dealings between genital parts. What about his sexual drive for the other, almost 60 000 hours of his existence on top of the world? It is difficult to imagine it was entirely sublimated by his smoking Maria Mancini cheroots and discussing the history of Western thought with Settembrini.

 Robert Musil, who was far more explicit about sexual needs in his own great unfinished novel *The Man without Qualities*—a novel that merits extended comparison with Mann's, not least since his protagonist Ulrich could almost be cousin to the naïve Hans Castorp in *The Magic Mountain*—wrote in his diary (Notebook 30): "One might criticise Th. Mann on the ground that he reminds one of a boy who has practised self-abuse and later becomes the head of a family. The knowledge of immorality and how the normal person comes to terms with it, this immorality—which has lost all danger and yet can be called to mind with a raised eyebrow—in the work of Thomas Mann can be traced back (virtually) only to that source. And what does his problem child, Castorp, do in all that time on the Magic Mountain? Obviously he masturbated! But M. removes the private parts from his characters as if they were plaster-of-Paris statues."

Mann, however, was most certainly alive to the possibilities of desire. Among the many cameo characters who populate the International Sanatorium Berghof—a microcosm of Europe itself— is Frau Salomon from Amsterdam, who gets "pleasure from displaying her lace underwear at examination." A coquette, in other words, who knows how to stimulate desire by withholding the possibility of its satisfaction or by feigning indifference to the effect she produces. I remember a couple of female patients from the Council of Europe who came to consult me in my practice in Strasbourg, and the evident pleasure they took at my look of surprise on glimpsing (as I prepared to examine them) their expensive Chantal Thomass brocaded silk underwear.

It had crossed my mind that I might even be a kind of Hans Castorp myself...

Multivit me

Americans like to think of themselves as rational, but many of my American friends, though perfectly healthy, are vitamin junkies. They owe this odd habit to Linus Pauling, who, though he was a brilliant chemist (and won the Nobel Prize for it), had a thing about vital amines: we certainly need them in traces to stay healthy, but the industry that has grown up around them is almost entirely useless. Some vitamins in excess will even make you ill.

Being part of a conversation

Franz Rosenzweig (1886-1929) isn't much read these days, which is a pity, since he was, like the much more famous Ludwig

Wittgenstein, a philosopher who knew the attractions of systematic thought in the German mode, and the danger of "objective" world-embracing rational schemes—such as Hegel's philosophy of the state. He concluded that philosophy without an existential impulse (as practised in universities) is a pretty vapid business, so he turned to dialogue—which is how philosophy had started. In 1921, the year in which his major work *The Star of Redemption* was published, he was commissioned by the Frommann publishing house to write an introduction to his philosophy for a lay audience. The result was a slim, ironic narrative about convalescence: *Understanding the Sick and the Healthy: A View of World, Man, and God*. The title is a pun on the German expression for common sense—"gesunder Menschenverstand"—and suggests that philosophy itself becomes sick when it abandons common sense.

Rosenzweig made a distinction between "logical" and "grammatical" thinking. The first has autistic traits: "it thinks for nobody else and speaks to nobody else." The advantage of this mode of thinking is that it allows a splendid isolation: it shelters the thinker from the mess, confusion and strife of the human throng and confers a kind of immunity against the risks and anxieties attendant on the thinking life. It alienates, but it allows a comfortable alienation. It glorifies substance and essence. And the philosophy it produces is attractive to rulers and administrators, since it suggests that the world is basically orderly and promises yet more order. It thrives behind sealed borders and on mountain tops, and in the lack of dissent from the streets. In fact, it has angelic qualities: angels are beings who can never surprise each other by doing something unexpected. In ordinary human terms it only ever *pretends* to have conversations. As Niklas Luhmann puts it, systems primarily have a relation with themselves and only marginally with external factors, including the so-called human element.

Years before them the great French diarist Joseph Joubert had identified the end-stopped effortless consequentialism of rational thinking at the time of the French Revolution. "Reason does not reason," he wrote. "It goes straight to the fact or outcome."

This kind of logical thinking, according to Rosenzweig, is the dominant feature of all academic philosophy, a manifestation of the disease he calls *apoplexia philosophia*. Philosophy cannot wait for wonder to resolve itself in the course of life. By interrogating what provokes wonder it removes itself, and the source of its wonder, from the flow of life. Any answers to its questions no longer have very much to say to the actual life in which they would be meaningful.

In fact, its answers are almost totally irrelevant to the everyday world. In the not-quite century since Rosenzweig had his revelation, we can see that his criticism of "logical" thinking now applies to other domains: much orthodox thinking, from risk management to sociology to economics, exhibits the same disconcerting attachment to an abstract world, while forgetting that language is only ever an idealisation of the real. That is why they are sometimes called "zombie" disciplines: they seem to be alive and functioning in a meaningful way, they quote names and numbers, they know the specialist literature; but it is obvious to everybody except their practitioners they have lost any connection to what matters. It may, conceivably, be happening in medicine too.

"Grammatical" thinking, on the other hand, emerges out of language. Speaking partners have a mouth, as well as ears. This means that grammatical thinking follows not the seating arrangements of logical systems but the shifting relations of a conversation—which has far-reaching implications for its development and outcome. People who discuss things participate in the mutual hope of saying something meaningful. Speaking "is bound by time and nourished by time and it neither can nor wants to abandon this element. It does not know in advance just where it will end. It takes its cues from others. In fact, it lives by virtue of another's life, whether this other is the one who listens to a story, answers in the course of a dialogue, or joins in a chorus." Thinking grammatically mean inviting others to join the conversation (a minimal, linguistic understanding of what is implied by the Biblical injunction to "love one's enemies"), realising what is at stake in a discussion, cultivating the faculty of listening, and not attributing an authority to facts determined by the logical mode of thinking that is greater than the actual problems confronted by people trying to live—and perhaps even think grammatically—in society. Patience takes on a new allure. Then it becomes clear what the Orcadian poet Edwin Muir meant: "The reason was, there was nothing there but faith."

When a life unfolds in time, Rosenzweig suggests, the wonder that provokes a person into thought finds its own resolution: the apprehension of self in the world that was the source of wonder becomes part of lived experience. That, as it happens, was also Socrates' definition of the *logos*—as a kind of love affair that cannot be read backwards. It entails a change of self.

NEEDLEPOINT

"What could be more important for such a young creature, one who is seriously ill, than to find a doctor who inspires trust at first sight?" asks the narrator of Ernst Weiss' novel in one of the more harrowing moments in *Georg Letham: Arzt und Mörder*, a child's life being at stake. "Many physicians have this ability. It can be seen in paediatric clinics when an exhausted tiny creature, in the midst of its suffering—suffering that can only be bewildering and thus all the more terrifying for it—will instantly stop all its wailing at the sight of a certain doctor, wipe away its tears with hands almost too weak to do anything, and with an indescribable expression of pure submissiveness, of courage, indeed of faith and even delight in the midst of distress, give itself up to the physician who, responding to the illness, not the gaze of the sick child, is preparing to examine it".

I recall that I had this ability too: V., our adolescent patient with leukaemia who had lost all her hair after chemotherapy, allowed only me, out of the twelve junior doctors on the roster at the Royal Hospital for Sick Children in Glasgow, to take blood or insert a cannula in her arm. She was perhaps a little smitten with me; and I was only too aware of this unsought-for complication as I quaked inwardly, armpits sodden with anxiety, unsure if her faith in me would survive a botched attempt to locate a vein on her much-punctured brachial fold. The presence of her anxious parents in the room didn't help. Never have I been more relieved that I could do something well. I was doing my next placement when I learned that she had died.

"Mein Gott, ich sehe!"—

"My God, I see!" is Thomas Mann's title for the key section of chapter five of *The Magic Mountain*, in which Hans Castorp on being confronted with the X-ray of his hand teeters imaginatively on the edge of his own grave. It is an exclamation which comes up at the moment of revelation, and recalls Socrates' discussion of the fitness of names in Cratylus when he attempts to match the soma ("body") with the sema ("grave"), and visualise the body metaphorically as the grave of the transparent soul. Hans has been unnerved by the realisation that X-rays can penetrate time as well as flesh and reveal us already as the skeletons to which we will be reduced at the end of our lives. Long before the advent of X-rays, the betrothed of Mr Venus, articulator of skeletons in Dickens's *Our Mutual Friend*, was unsettled by his profession: "I do not wish to regard myself, nor yet to be regarded, in that bony light".

H. T. Lowe-Porter, whose translations have been criticised over the years for their many howlers and distortions of sense, decided in her English version to use the ironic title "Sudden Enlightenment". She has obscured the verbal declamation Mann put in the mouth of his protagonist, but realised that the novelty of the section is all about the body being rendered not as bleeding flesh, as in the Renaissance tradition of écorché or flayed man, but as luminous presence.

Hypnosis and autonomy

It is a strikingly odd and disturbing fact that consciousness, which seems so central to human life, is a fluctuating and quite superficial phenomenon in respect of overall brain function: it can—inconveniently and at times unbeknown to the headspace in which it is thought to reside—be variously raised, lowered, duped, misplaced, even obliterated. Most people readily, indeed absentmindedly, slip into a trance, especially when performing routine activities such as driving; conversely actors, even Method actors, can snap out of even the most intense performance in a jiffy. Hypnosis ritualises some of these shifts in consciousness: it is no accident that hypnosis is so often associated with stage acts, and indeed has acquired a dubious reputation because of that association. Theatre audiences need to be kept in the dark in more ways than one, for hypnosis is a method of suggestion that works most effectively when the field of attention is filled with one sense activity only. The paralogical world of the spoken word then expands to become a hypnotised subject's entire mediated reality.

Autonomy is the great modern theme: oral cultures on the other hand were concerned with what could enter the ear and possess a person. Everything is caught by the ear at the same time; the visual mode by contrast is linear and successive. Yet the fear of possession has survived long into the modern era. And the more we look back at that era, which is still in historical memory, the more it appears that possession was a condition affecting the audience rather than the actors. If there was one deep reason why the Nazis had to do away with those they held to be their universal enemies, it was not because they themselves were hypnotised by a historical imperative. It was because the Nazis knew they themselves were *poseurs*, because they knew that the millennial history of the Jews, in particular, had been a long training in seeing through the presumptions and arrogance of all aspirations to power, especially those of a heroically hectoring Nobody who called himself the Leader.

A NEW COSMOLOGY

Paracelsus' statement, "And mark well this point, that all natural art and wisdom are given to men by the stars, and that nothing is excepted; that all things are given to us by the stars, and we are the students of the stars, and the stars are our teacher," finds its echo in Hölderlin's late ode *Chiron*: "And in the cool of the stars I learned, but/ Only the nameable."

I can only presume many pilgrims have walked in the cool of the stars and encountered that urgent question posed by an

Aramaic-speaking radical—rabbi, hasid and redeemer—in the oldest of the gospels: "Whom do men say that I am?"

Thinking about Lazarus

Jesus puts in a lot of work as a hak'am (*h-k-m* in the Semitic languages means "appoint, choose, judge", as in the Arabic term *hakim*, one of the ninety-nine names of Allah) in the New Testament, going around healing the lame and curing the sick with no medicines other than spittle and words. Thomas de Quincey observed that "As a hakim, Christ obtained that unlimited freedom of intercourse with the populace, which, as a religious proselytiser, he could never have obtained." Not once does he recommend to the halt and the harried that they should accept their lot and reconcile themselves to their suffering. As often as not, afflictions appear to be the devil's work.

He heals a man who has been lame from birth, telling him to stand up and walk off with his pallet; he cures a man with a withered hand; he gives sight to the blind, even to those blind from birth; he heals a woman who has been haemorrhaging blood for twelve years; he cures spinal deformities; he allows the mute to speak; he cures lepers. He issues commands and rebukes, and things happen. He cures a deaf-mute by putting his fingers into his ears, spitting and uttering the Aramaic imperative: *Ephphatha* ("Be opened!"). In another instance he uses a poultice of mud and saliva to cure a man who had been blind from birth. He touches people without being compelled to hold himself at a distance from their unclean bodies, and can even feel the curing power "come out of him". Mere contact with him or his garments in the marketplace is enough to impel cure: "All who had diseases pressed upon him to touch him" (Mark 3:10); and "as many as touched [the fringe of his clothes] were made well." (Mark 6:56). Jesus refrains from self-help, which is precisely the tenor of the heartless remark made by the elders as he hangs on the cross: "He saved others, but he is not able to save himself." (Mark 13:15).

Raising the dead would certainly have to be considered one of this charismatic wonder-worker's more unusual exploits: a triumph of evocation. It had been associated with other prophetic figures: both Elijah and Elisha came up with spectacular resuscitations, and charisma attached each to the latter's dry bones (2 Kings 13:20). Jesus raises Lazarus in front of a large crowd, with all the theatrical elements befitting such an extraordinary event. It is the third of three reanimations of the newly deceased mentioned in the New Testament.

Yet how much more difficult must Jesus have found it to provide something to assuage the never-ending human longing for explanation and consolation, and to still his own impending sense of abandonment.

"Go, your faith has healed you," he tells people—and is any other phrase more likely to generate a mood of expectation? Not only is a sick person cured, the world itself is poised for eschatological transformation, and the kingdom of heaven where "death shall be no more; neither shall there be mourning nor crying nor pain." (Revelation 21:4).

OUT OF DEPTH

The flatland is the name Thomas Mann chooses to describe the uninteresting life his main character Hans leads before he comes to join those "up there" on the Magic Mountain. Of course, the flatland is what we all seek to escape when we attempt to return to the "real" world: it extends across all our paper representations and media screens. As Edward Tufte writes, "nearly every escape from flatland demands extensive compromise, trading off one virtue against another...". Even our language, he observes, lacks the capacity to communicate "a sense of dimensional complexity." And that is what Hans does in the course of Mann's novel: he quits the conventional map on which the town of Davos is easy to find, and time itself is alternately swollen and emaciated. Hans' first three weeks at the sanatorium occupy half of the novel; and then the mountain loses a little of its contoured magic and engenders a kind of tedium in its turn.

The social contract

It is not so much that trust has disappeared from our lives, it is more that the forms of trust in a liberal society are mild ones, requiring only as much trust as is necessary to ensure the circulation of money, bonds, fiduciaries of all kinds: even a contract presupposes an element of trust though in bringing people together it also thrusts them apart—as adversaries upholding the bond of signature.

Magic made method

Oliver Wendell Holmes indulges in a bit of futurology. "Give us the luxuries of life and we will dispense with the necessities."

What we desire

Balzac's fable about modernity *La Peau de chagrin* (1831) is a disconcerting anticipation of the biological discovery of the telomere. Raphaël de Valentin, the young man on the make who serves as the story's hero, is on the verge of suicide after having ruined himself at the gaming tables. In extremis, he wanders into a kind of junk store and acquires an old donkey's skin inscribed with magical ciphers. The shagreen has the power to fulfil his deepest wishes but, as the mysterious shopkeeper warns him, at the expense of his life. "The compass of your days, manifest in that skin, will shrink according to the force and number of your desires, from whims to most extravagant notions."

Valentin enjoys the high life, and though he tries to forget about the skin it haunts the back of his mind: he even trains his servants to anticipate his wishes so as not to have to express them. But the repressed returns, for this scrap of skin has been satisfying desires he can barely acknowledge to himself. When his health starts failing, he is forced to come to terms with its shrinking, by which time it has of course shrunk to wafer size. He tries to rid himself of it, cut it, burn it, spoil it with chemicals, and he even tries to stretch it, but to no avail. Pauline, the love of his life, attempts desperately to do away with herself so that he won't desire her; but Valentin knows he has no grounds for resenting a bargain he once accepted so complaisantly. He cannot love her passively, or aspire to nirvana at this late hour; and he dies in her arms. It could even be argued that the shagreen itself has created a specific want. It certainly provides a kind of consummation.

Although Balzac's story has been interpreted as a morality tale about what happens to people who pursue worldly and social status it clearly has a more direct relationship to the unquenchable, unpredictable and unstable nature of human desire itself, which leads to our ruin *whether we bring it on or not*. Biologically speaking, it is not the skin that retracts but the telomere, those repetitive nucleotide sequences at the end of the chromosomes in most eukaryotic organisms (TTAGGG in humans). These sequences prevent chromosome deterioration and fusion during replication, and can be considered as disposable buffers: they protect the gene sequences from being unnecessarily truncated. Telomeres are replenished by an enzyme but over time become shorter. That is: telomeres serve a sacrificial function until the sacrificial resource itself dwindles away.

"A man has to die of knowing these things" as the old Egyptian papyrus fragment of Ptah-hotep states it, with some economy.

A COMEDY IN FOUR ACTS

Osip Mandelstam writes in his essay "The End of the Novel" that the Napoleonic era had caused the "stock value of the individual in history to rise in an extraordinary manner."

That stock value is never higher than in Chekhov's atmospheric plays where conversations in the dacha spill out into the poplar-lined meadow, and the whole scene is illuminated by figures chatting or sitting alone and cherishing their glass of wormwood liquor in the light of a provincial midsummer fading in the west. His plays are titrations of small moments, of lives and loves cloyed in frustrations but never entirely blighted. "Where is my past life," hankers Prozorov in *Three Sisters*, "oh, what had become of it—when I was young, happy and intelligent. When I had such glorious thoughts and visions, and my present and future seemed so bright and promising?" Chekhov's mature works are plays not of action or ideas, but of mood. Moods steeped in modern kinds of dissatisfaction. And all his characters have the air of saying something pertinent about the human condition by avoiding grand statements about the human condition. In fact, what they don't say contributes as much to the mood of his plays as what is said. Chekhov hints. He doesn't moralise. He evokes the passage of time: he is a connoisseur of the twilight moment between departure and nostalgia. And he leaves us—and his *dramatis personae*—to puzzle at the significance of what might be happening off-stage, like that enigmatic "sound of a breaking string" in *The Cherry Orchard*.

For all their fawning pretentiousness, social one-upping and foreknowledge of hope defeated, Chekhov loves these people. His loves them so much he turns them into musical instruments, such a gathering of pot-bellied cellos and sob-throated violins orchestrated for embarrassments, major and minor. All of Russia is their orchard, especially now that the day has just drawn in.

The soirée in *The Seagull* concludes as muted chamber music—*sotto voce*.

Bend or break

Now that "resilience" has become such a modish term including in ethics (even though until recently its primary meaning hardly applied to human beings at all), it is intriguing to realise that for Dr Johnson in one of his Rambler columns it meant almost the opposite of the flexible but obdurate quality it seems to have acquired. We don't simply cope these days, we are *resilient*; and we want to learn from those who refuse to give in or give up, even under conditions of extreme hardship and opposition.

In Column No. 111, "Repentance Stated and Explained",

Johnson enumerates the difficulties experienced by his contemporaries in lifting their intelligences to a true state of godliness and worries that some of the rules, "corrupted by fraud, or debased by credulity, have, by the common resiliency of the mind from one extreme to another, incited others to an open contempt of… the whole discipline of regulated piety." What he thinks of as "resiliency" is clearly a kind of perpetual swithering, or *vacillation*: this is what Friedrich Nietzsche, who stated more than once that he didn't believe in the "mythology" of the will, nonetheless called "a weak will", which he thought derived from a poor organisation of capacities and goals. He referred to it, in a manner not unlike Dr Johnson, as "oscillation and lack of gravity" (WP, 46).

This Puritan conception of the free-standing will—which clearly underwrites the modern notion of resilience—would have been alien to Thomas Aquinas, who believed that what we choose is implicit in the way our bodies are biased towards what is desirable. The will is how our existence turns us towards the intelligibility of things—which cannot be far from Dr Johnson's understanding of volition. We do not meaningfully recede from what we have in mind to do.

So perhaps we should be circumspect about psychologists who come talking resilience when what they actually mean is *self-reliance*. The fact that the term "resilience" has its true home in materials science—the realm of the insentient—perhaps advertises why it has become such an appealing concept-word for an age in which servitude dressed up as freedom of choice is the new capitalist mode: the important thing is that you respond to every situation that comes your way, whether good or bad, in the *optimal* manner. After all, the allied term "stress" itself entered the lexicon only in the 1930s, when the Hungarian endocrinologist Hans Selye started using it to describe the adverse circumstances (and their physiological and psychological effects) he was imposing on laboratory animals in some of his experiments. It had hitherto been used to describe the extreme forces applied to materials to determine their breaking point. Selye ultimately came to distinguish between "good stress" and "bad stress", as if realising that what seemed a neutral term actually had moral polarities.

In fact, as Hannah Arendt wrote, "events, by definition, are occurrences that interrupt routine processes and routine procedures." (You might think events are just "things that happen" but many philosophers and even cognitive scientists have developed careers showing that the ontological status of events barely fits into the regular humdrum of what we think of as "life".) People survive even dramatic events, although they are likely to be changed by them too. One of the definitions of the verb *resile* (now used almost exclusively by international lawyers) is "to return to the original position or state after being stretched or compressed." An elastic process is suggested. Better, surely, to have a sense of how an experience changes us than to aspire to bounce back to the status quo ante. Events that make us suffer are thresholds, and we have to cross them. That is what Dante's great poem is all about. On the other side of such experiences we are differently clothed.

But the central point about resilience is surely that it puts the onus entirely on the individual, rather than the organisation or larger society, to adapt. If you can't cope, then it must be because you are lacking this essential quality.

So let me mention another quality that outdoes resilience: the ability to overcome insults or *resurgence*...

A STILL LIFE

Over the years my fascination with the works of the Ostend master James Ensor has grown, what with his masquerades and mummeries, his baroque fantasies about sour herrings and odd Flemish words and his very visible intention to *épater les bourgeois* despite his own solidly bourgeois origins. He did have some odd and even slightly vulgar interests, not least in the tourist objects his parents sold in their curio shop but that hardly proved to be a disadvantage. He was an artist who shifted the boundaries of expressive decorum (in a very stuffy age) in a remarkable way, introducing caricature and satire into a broadly realistic tradition:

he even had a feeling for popular culture, showing revenge scenes where well-known Belgian figures get their comeuppance (with himself as Christ).

I wasn't familiar though with his strikingly realistic painting of his dead mother hanging in the Museum voor Schone Kunsten in his home city. His mother was eighty when she died in 1915 (he was 55), and she has the gone look of the defunct: sunken eyes, prominent nose, open mouth. In her clasped hands she holds a crucifix. Right of centre is an overdressed column with a statuette of the Virgin Mary, her head bent in mourning, but the entire foreground is occupied by a tray holding ten medicinal bottles and flasks. Their detailed contours and stoppers, and the way they catch the light makes it clear that these objects and their contents were the true focus of his mother's last days—the hope that some of these potions might keep her alive a few days more.

Rule of Three

In his spellbindingly erudite book *How to Kill a Dragon: Aspects of Indo-European Poetics*, the linguist Calvert Watkins surveys the threefold concept of medicine, as it appears in ancient Avestan, Vedic and Pindaric literature: there is a medicine of the knife, a medicine of plants, salves and potions and a medicine of holy formulas or verbal incantations. These three functions provided the three types of curative treatments before it was ever presumed that soul and body were separate entities.

While medicine and surgery have flourished under modern conditions, it has been a long time since anyone had her ailments banished by a recital of a Rigvedic hymn to the healing divinities. Even the talking cure is not what it was. Jacques Lacan would charge you 500 francs for ten minutes, and not say a word the whole time. He too had a tripartite scheme which accounted for the more restricted sphere of human subjectivity: inextricably linked with the ego drive of the Imaginary and the structured language of the Symbolic was the Real, an irreducable realm of non-meaning.

"The real," he told a group of Italian journalists in 1974, "is the difference between what works and what doesn't work. What works is the world. The real is what doesn't."

How to deal with epidemics

Now and again society gets visited by the cognitive plague. This compels all citizens, those nodes of sovereign consciousness, to assume that doctors have a hidden agenda because they explicitly cultivate a fiduciary relationship with them as patients; and apply a Cartesian strategy of suspicion. Then they discover that the warm friendly atmosphere they used to cherish no longer exists, and lament that "the old-fashioned general practitioner, with whom you could have a conversation, is nearly extinct" (Sheila Hale). There is no escape from this tension though, as Ernest Gellner wrote, "many are offered on the market."

Warmth will always come creeping back in when money is the coin of trust, because the force needed to see what is real in the Kingdom of Large Numbers can only be redeemed with love for the individual person.

Moral hyperinflation

One day some brilliant young sociologist or medical historian will have a field day analysing the change of tone in the house organ of the British Medical Association over the twenty years of what have been my mixed professional experience of medicine. Serenely, superciliously confident in the early 1980s, the *British Medical Journal* of the 1990s exhibited a new bullish, sometimes hubristic tone; and the editorials and commentaries stacked at the front of the journal were clearly modelled on those of *The Economist*. But a funny thing had happened to medicine on the way to the marketplace. The great sin had become paternalism. The patient was idealised. "Care" became the new orthodoxy.

Suddenly it became a familiar experience to encounter

personal articles in which doctors donned sackcloth and ashes and, flagellating themselves withal, confessed their sins in public. Had medical idealism gone to the dogs? No, it was just that doctors had imploded under the strain of being moral paragons with one foot in the moribund British civic religion while aiming to maximise gain like any rational *homo œconomicus*. And then the monstrous Harold Shipman heaved into view, nurtured by some "hideous sense of power" in Oscar Wilde's words, like one of those sinister Victorian poisoners immortalised in Madame Tussaud's waxworks…

SEEPAGE

In an interview the retired pathologist and author F. Gonzalez-Crussi states that whenever he was called on to perform a post mortem he would always place a drape over the patient's head.

As he comments, keeping up appearances in this way is an odd thing to do since the person is gone and the cadaver has no emotions or projects—its bodily substance may even be in a state of advanced decomposition. But it seems to be a pathologist's tradition. One of the earliest Dutch group portraits of anatomists, "The Anatomy Lesson of Dr. Willem van der Meer" by Michiel van Miereveld, commissioned by the surgeon's guild of Delft in 1617, shows a partially eviscerated cadaver with a ribbon of gauze over his eyes.

When the interviewer asks if he would have felt disturbed to have seen the faces of those he was dissecting Gonzalez-Crussi has the perfect reply: he doesn't know, because he always covers their faces.

Insofar as photographs are post mortem relics too (although their subjects may be alive a while longer), Roger Grenier writes that the American photographer Lisette Model used to lock up her dark room archives at night so that the souls of the photographed wouldn't wander through the studio and haunt her in her sleep.

Future improvements

A friend in Geneva showed me his copy of the pioneering work *The Statistical Account of Scotland*, in which Sir John Sinclair (1754–1835) supervised the first attempt to give an accurate portrait, in 21 volumes, of the conditions pertaining in his native land. As in Germany and the Scandinavian countries, churchmen were instrumental in collecting the information: communications from ministers of the various parishes provided the material for the account. "The idea I annex to the term is an inquiry into the state of a country, for the purpose of ascertaining the quantum of happiness enjoyed by its inhabitants, and the means of its future improvement; but as I thought that a new word might attract more public attention, I resolved on adopting it, and I hope it is now completely naturalised and incorporated with our language." This political arithmetic gave rise to the notion of society as a form of nature which would require light management only, since it like the larger nature ("all that is") ought to be able to regulate itself. But the numerical table still required to be developed as an instrument of persuasion.

Sir John Sinclair represented Caithness in the House of Commons. Robert Burns wrote to him about his rational statistical enterprise. It was at Sinclair's suggestion that the British government issued Exchequer Bills to avoid ruin in 1793, and adopted the "loyalty loan" of eighteen million pounds in order to prolong the war against the French. He is the subject of Henry Raeburn's magnificent romantic portrait in tartan breeks hanging in the National Gallery of Scotland. Some of his land was emptied of tenants and made over to sheep.

A bare quarter-century later legislators were trying to establish not the "quantum of happiness" but the "spot of sickness"—although our current legislators seem to have swung around to investigating the former again.

The last act

Edith Cavell's last words were carved on the plinth of her statue in the late 1920s, "when wartime hatreds had receded," asserts Susan Pedersen in a review of Diana Souhami's biography of the Britain's "Second Most Famous Nurse." In fact, the release in 1928 of Herbert Wilcox's silent film *Dawn*, with Sybil Thorndike in the starring role, added heat to the debate about her role in helping Allied soldiers to escape from Belgium and stirred dormant consciences on both sides of the former divide. It is a curiosity of literary history that Gottfried Benn, the German expressionist poet, was present at the execution in his official capacity as surgeon major to the German army in Brussels: he confirmed Cavell's death, closed her eyes and laid her in the coffin.

These details come from the eyewitness account "How Miss Cavell was shot" ("Wie Miss Cavell erschossen wurde") which Benn published, thirteen years after the event, in the evening edition of the National-Zeitung on 22 February 1928. It appears he was stung to write the piece partly by the controversial execution in Boston of the anarchists Sacco and Vanzetti—a *cause célèbre* in Europe and one which a liberal Berlin paper had called a "judicial murder", likening it to the German execution of Cavell—and also to refute the fallacious suggestion in the film that Cavell had been dispatched with a "mercy shot".

Although not unsympathetic to Cavell, Benn justified the execution as a historical necessity: "world history is not the basis of happiness and the posts of the Pantheon are smeared with the blood of those who act and then suffer, as demanded by the law of life." His tone is an odd mixture of Prussian coolness and appeal to the new Weimar feminism: "How is the shooting of Miss Cavell to be judged? It was all quite official and legal. She acted as a man and was punished by us as a man. She worked actively against the German army and she was crushed by this army. She had entered into the war and the war annihilated her. The French, too, shot a woman as a spy. I believe that today's woman not only understands this outcome but demands it."

Disobligingly, Thea Sternheim, wife of the dramatist Carl, who lived in Brussels at the time and knew Benn well, confessed to her diary (*Tagebücher* 1903-1971, published in five volumes in 2002) that she found Benn a bit too gimlet-eyed: he saw the execution with the "frightful objectivity of a doctor cutting up a corpse." Benn's effortless grasp of the first-hand report as an exercise in style prompted the left-wing writer and pioneer roving reporter Egon Erwin Kisch to write an article a year later which concluded: "Gottfried Benn is a... snob who has no idea about the world, but treats it [aber sie handelt]"—i.e. in the manner of a doctor.

Better to do good than just talk about doing good

This instruction brings us back to the peculiarity of the Western tradition, in its beginnings with Socrates, founder of the metaphysical tradition that gives precedence to the declarative sentence, over its imperative or ostensive forms (as in Chinese culture). Which must be why we're *still* talking about doing good.

William Blake, in another context, talked about "Doing Good in Minute Particulars." It is a peculiarly French foible to *talk* about doing good: I'm constantly struck, living in the country, by the gulf between the brilliance of the analyses of how to make solidarity meaningful, and the rather hopeless attempts to ensure that the social glue stays sticky. When a writer declares "I care about the life of every human being" then it hardly has to be said that "care" is an empty concept. France generally suffers from an overinvestment in the intellect and lack of spontaneity in social relations. Caring might be intellectually unenthralling, but patients never cease to surprise you. One old Alsatian patient I had used to tell me about his wartime experiences, when he shivered daily in fear for his life—as a *German* combatant in a Russian prisoner of war camp.

As Robert Pinsky puts it in his poem *The Questions*: it's no good "this new superfluous caring," you have to be someone "who learns that the janitor// Is Mr. Woodhouse; the principal is Mrs. Ringleven; the secretary/ In the office is Mrs. Apostolacos; the bus driver is Ray."

The philosopher as hospital porter

During the Second World War, Ludwig Wittgenstein, unhappy at being confined to his rooms in Cambridge, was invited by John Ryle to do voluntary work as an orderly at Guy's Hospital where almost nobody knew he was a famous philosopher. He was responsible for bringing batches of medications to the wards, where, as John Ryle's wife said, he used to advise patients not to take them. He later worked in the dispensary, mixing simple ointments for dermatological application. In those largely pre-pharmaceutical days, one wonders which particular drugs might have aroused Wittgenstein's scepticism.

Curing fantasies, purging follies

The famous etching by Martin Droeshout, which was published in London circa 1620, shows the interior of an apothecary's shop, with the doctor (Dr Panurgus) in his robes using a dose of "sagesse" to purge a "rude Rusticall," who voids lots of little fools beneath the close-stool on which he is perched, while a fashionably dressed man and woman (holding a squirrel on a leash) wait to be treated; on the right a young gallant with his head in a furnace is having his fads and fancies steamed right out of him. They emerge in a cloud at the top, and include playing cards, dice, a backgammon-board, pipes, a violin, masks, a plumed hat, a boy flying a kite, and a man with wings strapped to his shoulders. In an uncanny way the young man with his head in the furnace resembles contemporary patients being introduced headfirst into the birdcage of an MRI (magnetic resonance imaging) apparatus, for T1- and T2-weighted sequences in various planes, so that his chimeras and crochets might be plain to all.

Somewhere in the shop will be an ancient lodestone, which

was the common term for magnetite; it is from the modern understanding of electromagnetism that MRI was developed, using various intermittent gradients applied over the constant watery volume of a patient's body.

BLINDED

One of the disturbing implications of James Le Fanu's book *The Rise and Fall of Modern Medicine* (1999) is that the now rigorous enforcement of peer-reviewing and double-blinding (the "gold" standard) has not been accompanied by anything like the results which British medicine, specifically general practice, saw in its Golden Age (c. 1945-75). It was actually more of a free-for-all empiricism—trial and error, self-regulation and open studies, underwritten by a widely accepted if not always explicit ethic of cognition—which produced the therapeutics and medical products that were to bestow on medicine, for the first time in its history, a reputation for efficacy. When the sulpha drugs and penicillin were developed in the 1940s, it was obvious to everybody in the wards that they worked: controlled studies were not required. The ingress of epidemiology and statistics is thus a sign of the *decadence* of clinical medicine.

FREUD & CO.

At the New York World's Fair in 1939, Edward Bernays, nephew of Sigmund Freud, created a future vision of a world in which the consumer appeared to be king: his futurama was to be given the even uglier name Democracity. It introduced the American public, just before the war in distant Europe, to television, the early fax machine, nylons, fluorescent lighting, long-distance phone calls, and an underwater Salvador Dali exhibit starring a troupe of half-naked mermaids.

Bernays' feeling for social choreography was strongly influenced by his uncle's pessimistic view of human nature:

humans are simply too irrational to be entrusted with the full rights of citizenship, as classically understood. What he had brought with him from the old continent was a notion first dreamed up by the Viennese civil service and put into service after 1870 by the Germans, a new doctrine called *Kulturpolitik*, which converted the arts into instruments of national self-assertion. The four years of the Great War, during which President Wilson annulled many basic freedoms guaranteed by the constitution, made it clear on the other side of the Atlantic how easily forces could be set in motion to guarantee uniformity: the state is never more powerful than when at war. After he had graduated from Cornell and established his own PR company (or "propaganda business", as it was then called), Bernays increasingly began to sound like Dostoevsky's Grand Inquisitor: this was a man who knew what he was doing and explained why he did it with brutally disarming frankness. Managing perceptions and opinions was going to be even more necessary in a supposedly "free" democracy than an autocracy. Product advertising which, until about 1920, had tended to focus on attributes and quality now related goods to individual needs, and set about manufacturing those needs as well. Bernays saw that citizenship would be a much more manageable concept if the citizen could be encouraged to be a consumer and go in ignorance of consumption's ugly sister, production. By the year 2000, this deeply conservative if not downright cynical way of thinking had evolved into the marketing focus group technique that shaped the "politics" of the Clinton and Blair years. Give the people what they want but make sure you drill them to know what they want first! PR is now the means used by the rich and powerful to communicate with the rest of society.

In 1984, in his mid-nineties, Bernays finally achieved widespread celebrity as the father of marketing techniques and spin. The man who had "orchestrated the commercialisation of society", persuaded a generation of American women to start smoking cigarettes (which he termed "torches of freedom"), polished the image of two presidential hopefuls, helped the United Fruit Company and the US government topple the elected president of Guatemala in 1954 and whose 1928 book *Propaganda* was unreservedly admired by Joseph Goebbels, was invited on the David Letterman show.

Letterman: "Doctor, tell me again what the doctor is...? What are we dealing with here...? You're the father of public relations..."

Bernays (slowly and deliberately): "Well, what we're dealing with really is the concept that people will believe me more if you call me Doctor."

Studio audience: [thunderous applause].

Mythic physiology of the emotions

To say your heart *goes out* has a surprisingly pre-psychological, almost Aztec ring to it. The unconditionally faithful Cordelia in *King Lear* refuses to heave hers into her mouth (which is where the Egyptians thought it ought to be). The pure Sufi heart (*qalb*) has the power of sight. The Pietists also had hearts with eyes, and mother-hearts and heart-friends too. Rousseau's heart spoke to other hearts.

You surely wouldn't confuse the organ which has its reasons of which Reason knows nothing with blood surging through the aorta, would you?

Then they wrote the rules

After the magnificent, brutal, peremptory violence of the epics had faded from ancient Greece, and the heroic age was over and done with, what was left was the gift of madness, expressed through prophecy, song and the doings of doctors, as listed in Plato's *Phaedrus*.

Autonomy and crisis

The most extended saying of Heraclitus that has come down to us (preserved by Sextus Empiricus) concludes by insisting that humans "are oblivious of what they do awake, just as they are forgetful of what they do asleep". This might suggest a rather arrogant assurance on the part of the philosopher, who alone has stepped out of the human condition and into the clarity and brilliance of universal consciousness, whence he observes other humans as sleepwalkers with only enough surplus intelligence to make sure they don't collide with legions of other sleepy people on their way back to bed. It is like Jesus's saying—"forgive them, for they know not what they do"—but with wraparound cognitive force. These sleepwalkers dream when asleep, and then wake up but continue to dream, only now with added sensory input.

And yet Heraclitus' paradoxical saying describes what we truly know of the human condition, especially its physical part. Our lives are run for us not by servants but by processes into which we have no insight, other than when they go wrong—and even then, hardly any. We are in a very curious sense *possessed*, if not by demons. It takes a crisis to make us realise that an awful lot of our lives takes place out of the reach of intelligence or even bodily sensation. This observation led another, much later philosopher, Schopenhauer, to remark that it is only when the great flow of unconscious vegetative life is disrupted that we take notice of the state we are in. And he gave the philosophy of opposites a metaphysical edge. "I therefore know of no greater absurdity," he writes, "than that absurdity which characterizes almost all metaphysical systems: that of explaining evil as something negative. For evil is precisely that which is positive, that which makes itself palpable; and good, on the other hand, to wit all happiness and all gratification, is that which is negative, the mere abolition of a desire and extinction of a pain."

For Schopenhauer, justice, freedom and health are all *empty* concepts, merely vestigial in relation to their opposites.

A word aside

That was no digression, my long-winded friend: clinically speaking it was a *herniation*.

A COMMON CAUSE

Very few guild monopolies still exist—indeed they cannot exist under the egalitarian conditions that characterise market society. For about a century medicine was one of the few modern professions to be *sacramentally* distinguished from other walks of life, a privilege that only one or two individual practitioners ever enjoyed—and that precariously—in a more traditional society, where prestige and power were directly proportional to the distance of doctor from patient in the manner of the old priestly hierarchies.

Having for a time embraced the cause of those it served, now medicine appears to be changing into a service industry, if not a lip-service industry.

DEPENDENCIES

Jan de Vries' volume *The Industrious Revolution* turns our gaze away from the almost universally accepted dogma that the Industrial Revolution was solely responsible for a "supply-side" growth in consumption within the market economy of the nineteenth century. While the latter made it possible to boost productivity to levels hitherto unsuspected, and thus fulfil the desire of ordinary people for a better standard—and style—of living, it didn't create demand.

Vries shows that, long before the first factories appeared in Lancashire, men and women, first in the Netherlands and then in the British Isles and British America, were beginning to fill their homes with Delft, tobacco goods and linen, muslins and cotton cloths, which were lighter and brighter than the traditional woollen ware. Tobacco, soap, candles, printed fabrics, spirits and beer were being bought or consumed in the last years of the eighteenth century faster than the population was growing. England was a "nation of shopkeepers" a century before Napoleon popularised the phrase, with labouring families in cities acquiring their entire diet from local "grocery shops".

By 1711 authors at *The Spectator* expected to be "served up" every morning with a pot of tea, which Dr Johnson so much enjoyed that he once drank seventeen cups in a sitting. Richard Collins painted a famous family group in 1727 all enjoying a bowl of tea. Soon loose-leaf tea became cheaper, and democratised. Moralists were appalled at the amount of tea-drinking among the lower classes. The long eighteenth century—between 1650 and 1850—was when luxury triumphed, and writers such as Bernard Mandeville and Adam Smith dared to suggest that the desire for a better material life might stimulate the economy. With the new mercantile age came the imperative to shed traditional barriers against luxury and to elaborate philosophical justifications for excess.

The British Empire, it would therefore appear, was brought into existence in order to satisfy a drug rush: the good squires of letters and ladies of uncertain means were all high on sucrose, nicotine and alkaloids.

A FATAL LETHARGY

Fear of death is our common dread; but fear of not being dead at the time of the disposal of our corpses is another dread with a surprisingly long history—legend has it that the philosopher Duns Scotus having lapsed into a coma was buried alive in Cologne. Being buried alive has sometimes been a judicial if cruel punishment, as mentioned by Dante and depicted as a torture garden of legs thrashing the air by Doré in one of his engravings for the Inferno. Jan Bondeson, in his book *Buried Alive*, even suggests that it is our most primal fear. The ancient Romans, it is reputed, washed cadavers with boiling water before dressing them for the pyre. Another tradition has it that a finger was amputated before the corpse was burned. This may well be the origin of the undertaker's assistant or croque-mort, a popular figure of stage and song from the early eighteenth century, whose task it was to break the large toe of the deceased. (In French argot, "croquer" also means "to get rid of", which suggests that the croque-morts might simply have had other business with the dead.) Archaeologists researching a site where victims of the 1720-22 plague in Marseilles were buried found cadavers where pins had been stuck into the large toe to ascertain whether the corpses were truly dead.

All of which suggests that the famous *facies hippocratica*, a diagnostic description of death left in the corpus of his writings by Hippocrates—"the nose sharp, the eyes sunken, the temples fallen in, the skin of the face hard, stretched and dry, and the colour of the face pale or dusky"—has not always been a reliable index of portending death. In the eighteenth century it began to become common for death to be affirmed when the sense organs failed to react to stimulation. Jean-Jacques Bruhier (and his naturalist friend Buffon) devised some surgical tests: incision, needling, scarifying, as well as the application of hot iron or electrical current. Icard, a physician who specialised in death rites, invented a thanatograph, a compressive instrument which could be applied to the lips or other part of the skin. In the living person, the ischaemic trace produced by the clamp rapidly become irrigated again; in the dead person, it remained wrinkled, like parchment. Applying heat to the skin created a blister: Ott's sign indicated death if the blister was not serous but dry. There was even a macabre tossing test, which calls to mind Goya's famous painting "The Straw Manikin": the test called for four able-bodied persons to place the corpse in the middle of a canvas sheet and toss it in the air for half-an-hour. Bruhier suggests that many lives had been saved by this "épreuve du bernement et du saut." There were proposals for paracentesis of the thorax, so that the attending physician could lay his finger directly on the heart of the diseased, and thus confirm its non-contractility. (This technique now forms one of the heroic emergency strategies designed to *preserve* life in the event of cardiac arrest.) Icard wanted to inject a colorant into the heart and see whether it diffused into the eye. More poetically, mirrors, feathers and flames were all used to see whether the breath of life still animated the thoracic cage. But all of these inventive tests yielded to the power of electricity, which was first used to stimulate the muscles of a dead person in 1794. Not putting electricity into the body but measuring the body's own intrinsic electrical activity saw the development of the electrocardiogram in the 1920s, followed by the encephalogram, the flatness of which was one of the official Harvard criteria for recognising brain death in 1968.

Perhaps the burgeoning of medical tests was part of the problem, and the colossal success of Bruhier's "Dissertation on the Uncertainty of the Signs of Death" enjoyed a vogue and was translated into many languages. The nineteenth century, the era of positivism and materialism, saw the most florid wave of this fear of being buried alive, as illustrated by Antoine Wiertz's painting *L'inhumation précipitée*. Hans Christian Andersen, Arthur Schopenhauer, Frédéric Chopin and Wilkie Collins were some of the more famous persons to make stipulations in their wills that measures were to be taken after their ostensible death in order to confirm that they were "really" dead. "When she got old and ill my grandmother grew frightened of being buried alive and she constantly asked for assurance that she would be given an autopsy," writes Hubert Butler in his essay "Aunt Harriet". Aunt Harriet wasn't alone in this fear. The French historian Jules Michelet had a terror of premature burial, not only for himself for those close to him. He had the coffin of his first wife and father exhumed, and ordered the body of his Uncle Narcisse to be scarified before entombment. Rigor mortis, which sets in a few hours after death, was never sign enough. From being a slightly wonky craze, taphephobia became something of a moral panic. A German military doctor suggested in the early nineteenth century that as many as one in three inhumations were of not yet dead persons. It became common for wills to request doctors to open arteries and cut soles with scalpels in order to make doubly sure. In Germany, lying-in became an activity not just for expectant mothers: at the Hospitals for the Dead bodies could be left for several days until the unmistakable signs and smell of decomposition had set in. This was an Alsatian speciality: the mortuary at the Hôpital civil in Strasbourg was still admitting the newly defunct until the Second World War. Rings were attached to the fingers so that the deceased could pull a bell for assistance. Rare indeed were the summonses. It was even possible to be sent six feet under in a coffin fitted with an overground alarm bell. And it wasn't just the Germans. In 1905 the British social reformer (and anti-vaccinationist) William

Tebb published a book *Premature burial, and how it may be prevented* which gave details on a couple of several hundred cases of near live burial, and 149 actual cases: Tebb stipulated in his will that "unmistakable evidence of decomposition" was to be apparent before he was cremated.

Of course, part of the horror of the situation, imaginatively speaking, is that there are so few accounts of persons who have been buried and come back to tell the tale: this is the stuff of Edgar Allan Poe's story *The Premature Burial*. Illustrious Victorians took extraordinary precautionary measures to ensure Lazarus experiences would not be theirs. And of course, the most famous revenant of all is Jesus of Nazareth, who lay in the tomb for three days and came back from the dead only to disappear again, this time without trace.

The Milky Way

Steven Connor talks in his astonishing encyclopaedia of the epidermis *The Book of Skin* about being brought up in Britain "during the orgiastically lactic years that followed the Second World War."

There was surely little that was orgiastic about those years (not until the 1960s at any rate), but they were certainly lactic. I remember the half-pint cartons of milk handed out to us in primary school during the morning break, and the curious square-shaped electric cars which delivered the milk to the houses in our street every morning, two or three glass bottles sitting on the doorstep, all of them sealed with aluminium caps and bearing an inch or two of thick yellow cream above the milk.

The little phrase

In the spring of 1880, the nine-year-old Marcel Proust returned from the Bois de Boulogne after a walk with his parents and had his first severe asthmatic crisis. His more robust younger brother Robert described how even their experienced physician father Dr Achille-Adrien Proust, who was a professor of public health and served in the French ministry as Inspector-General of Sanitary Services, feared for his son's life, so severe was his "crise de suffocation." Marcel would suffer similar episodes most springs and summers, and had developed stridor and suffocation attacks every time he went to the countryside around his father's village of Illiers, which is called Combray in his great novel. By the age of 14, he was being sent instead to the seaside (Dieppe, Cabourg, Trouville) or to mountain spas for the summer recess. He had one or two dramatic train journeys later in his life, even after (or perhaps because) the carriages had been fumigated on his orders.

Having acknowledged the role of tree and grass pollens in the onset of his symptoms, Proust expanded the list to include all kind of irritants: dust, smells, noise and even the wind. "The acrid smell of your laundry causes unnecessary coughing fits," he complained to his servant Céleste Albaret. "I have coughed 3000 times." He forbad her from using naphthalene mothballs in the cupboards, asked her not to wax the parquet, prohibited coal fires, disinfected his mail with formol and wore gloves for working in bed, avoided overperfumed visitors altogether and insisted on the others smearing their nostrils with an ointment of purified niaouli (*Melaleuca quinquenervia*). Procured under its proprietary name "Rhino-goménol" by Mme Verdurin in *A la Recherche du Temps Perdu*, this was a nasal decongestant and antiseptic that was widely used in the early part of the twentieth century.

Once he had become an "asthmatique", Marcel could spend all his time inhabiting the paradox of his isolation from the world in the 3000-page life-consuming epic he was creating. He was writing short subordinate clauses embedded in an elegant syntax that caught the saccadic rhythm of his dyspnoea: the most ignoble or self-indulgent life was worthy because it would ultimately be lost. The ascetic impulse to sacrifice his life to art was a guarantee of this nominal faith in its totality. That was all anybody might hope to "regain." It is extraordinary that hardly anybody remembers that this key writer was the son of Dr Adrien Proust, one of France's leading experts on the mysterious condition of "aboulia" or lack of will which, along with the "perpetual sensation of fatigue", constituted that new disease of modernity: neurasthenia. In 1897, Proust's father even published a textbook on the condition called *L'Hygiène du neurasthénique*: it fascinated his sickly son. Although Marcel's masterpiece provides precious little detail about his distinguished father, doctor-brother Robert or even his own hermetic existence coughing in his cork-lined apartment, it is pervaded by what might be called *the clinical attitude*: a kind of diagnostic objectivity that underwrites the subjectivity and introspection. He even fancied that he had an intuitive understanding of nervous disorders himself.

"Even when he was not thinking of the little phrase, it existed latent in his mind on the same footing as certain other notions without material equivalent, such as our notions of light, of sound, of perspective, of physical pleasure, the rich possessions wherewith our inner temple is diversified and adorned. Perhaps we shall lose them, perhaps they will be obliterated, if we return to nothingness. But so long as we are alive, we can no more bring ourselves to a state in which we shall not have known them than we can with regard to any material object, than we can, for example, doubt the luminosity of a lamp that has just been lit, in view of the changed aspect of everything in the room, from which even the memory of the darkness has vanished…" (*Swann in Love*).

Proust was able to write such an "infinite" novel, somebody once said, by constantly harping on the adjective "little": the little clan of the Verdurins, Swann's little eye for the ladies, the little expanse of yellow wall in Vermeer's painting of Delft. And of course, the little madeleine—"la petite madeleine." It is out of this tiny detail of perception that he creates a 3000-page disquisition on the unity of selfhood, the unity which a crumb of madeleine dunked in a cup of herbal tea reveals is lost.

The breath of life

The modern nursing custom of stopping up the orifices (rectum and vagina) and putting a roll or bolster under the chin of a newly deceased person was already laid out in the practical instructions of the Mishnah—the first significant written collection of existing Jewish oral traditions—to separate the dead from the living. "They tie the cheeks" (Shabbat 23:5) if the mouth gapes open, "and they stop his bowels", the whole procedure being less concerned with the fact that the dead person should not emit the odours and sounds of decomposition than "that air should not enter." The entire corpse was to be entirely sealed off from the physical world except—intriguingly enough—for the ear, the conduit of belief, which "cannot hear because it is forbidden to speak in the presence of the body." (Berakhot 3:1).

Meanwhile, the body would also be washed and dressed, and its hair and nails trimmed, which are all acts of continuity with the living, and certainly familiar to modern nurses too.

Personal Jesus

It was Jean-Jacques Rousseau who introduced the modern fashion for baring the soul. "I know my own heart... I am made unlike anyone I have ever met. I even venture to say that I am like no one in the whole world. I may be no better, but at least I am different." Protestants had kept diaries to show the progress of their soul, in order to detail the dangers to which it had been exposed to and narrowly escaped; Rousseau took his stand on honesty, whatever the cost it might entail for himself and others, and became the first exhibitionist. What had formerly been a sin became a glory. And from baring the soul it was but a slip of the hand to ripping bodices, and far more extravagant kinds of perversions and cruelties; the Marquis de Sade told his wife that all his inspiration came from Rousseau. And our modern revolutionaries use honesty to oppose culture itself. Yet Rousseau was a faithful follower of the Christian conviction that, irrespective of our birth and station, we are all spiritually naked in the world.

The vagrant uterus

Searchers were paid to bury the dead of London, and they kept laconic and mysterious sounding records of the apparent cause of death. Their terms included "Affrighted", "Grief", "Itch", "Piles", "Planet", "Rising of the Lights" and "Mother". This last was often recorded as a cause of death in Shakespeare's time, being an anglicising of the matrix or uterus, which had been on its travels around the body. When Lear says "O, how this mother swells up toward my heart!" he is talking about *hysterica passio*, which was thought to be accompanied by symptoms of choking and shortness of breath. The searchers could only have had this knowledge on hearsay.

Hysteria is now considered to be a curious historical legacy— or as some say "a catch-all junk diagnosis"—not least on account of the variety of its possible manifestations.

After virtue

In 2002, I attended a symposium in London called "The Virtuous Doctor" which sought according to its organiser to explore "the character of moral agents" as a way of responding to the perceived crisis about medical standards of practice and falling morale in the profession. It seemed clear enough to me that the pursuit of wealth under market conditions had already destroyed the implicit system of values that made it possible for general practice to become a respected occupation in the first place, not least stable social relationships, jobs for life, and the assumption of trust in others. To try to define the virtuous practitioner was closing the stable doors when the horse had bolted. Even then it might be thought that markets need a degree or uprightness and decency in order to function well and be efficient, even as they are bound to undermine those virtues. Adam Smith thought "natural sympathy" would set limits on what persons would be willing to do in the pursuit of self-interest. Yet perhaps only a thinker coming from the poor but educated society of eighteenth-century Scotland where sympathy had been inculcated between the classes, in other words as a cultural ritual, could make the mistake of thinking it to be *natural*. (It is still a feature of the country's civil life.) As Nietzsche would have told him: "When one has a virtue, a real virtue, a complete virtue [...], one is its victim!"

The rather shocking irony about this symposium was that its organiser wanted to find a way of quantifying the virtues, as if they could be checklisted—as so many "quality parameters." This was tantamount to saying: give me a mechanism and I'll show you a moral! This of course was where the research money lay. The virtues were being ticked off as part of a portfolio career plan. That, more than anything else, suggested how unsuited we were to talk about them at all. We were either cynically at work debasing the coinage, or like the characters in Jack Womack's SF-novel *Elvissey* who all hanker to be virtuous although nobody can quite recall what the virtues *are*.

Then I had a terrible thought: might the future, in fact, be a nightmare of virtuousness? The virtues come from the same place as the notion of the virtual. They derive from the Latin *virtus*, meaning potency or efficacy, especially in the sense of male force. "Virtual" seems to have come about in the early fifteenth century to designate something that exists in effect, though not in fact. Now we can plainly see how moral qualities that don't exist can be made to appear to exist. Which is precisely what that eminent philosopher Alasdair MacIntyre called "the masquerade of the virtues".

I went back to France nourishing the dark thought that once the middle classes endeavour to look virtuous, vice takes on an unmistakable allure. "Let not virtue seek/ Remuneration for the thing it was!" as Shakespeare warned (in *Troilus and Cressida*).

The radical votive

"Goya in gratitude to his friend Arrieta for the skill and great care with which he saved his life in his acute and dangerous illness, suffered at the end of 1819, at the age of seventy-five years." So reads the caption.

When you have understood the radical force of Goya's ex-voto *Self-portrait with Dr Arrieta* (1820)—the theatrical sickbed scene showing his attentive personal physician, the said Dr Eugenio García Arrieta, cradling him in the crook of his left arm while lifting up with the right a glass of potion for him to drink—then you may be ready to concede with the French novelist J.M.G. Le Clézio, son of a surgeon, that there is "no art but only Medicine." Goya's portrait—from his years of exile in Bordeaux—of Dr Arrieta, who is both nurse and doctor, is a picture of tact and skill: if it is not Goya's own masterpiece it is surely the finest portrayal of a physician in art.

Lit from below, the painting reveals an even more intimate etymology: a *conspiracy*, which etymologically and in a neutral sense means a "breathing together": you can almost hear the patient's laboured gasps for air. Goya is in a sad, stricken state: maintaining his station only with difficulty, his head tilted back and his fingers restlessly plucking at the white sheet on the bedstead pulled over his lower body. He seems to be a man exhausted and resigned, a man who has closed his eyes and given up on life. Goya could even be an elderly Christ supported by a blue-frocked angel. This is the painter looking back from the edge of the grave, his face as grey as death. But he resists his death-wish, if we can call it that. For this singular painting is that singular thing, an Enlightenment pietà.

Instead of abandoning his almost moribund patient (*desahucio* or evicted from the realm of the living), Dr Arrieta has inspired the first truly modern artist to resist those old temptations: despondency and despair. He looks not at the viewer, but meditatively, resolutely, into the half-distance at bottom right. His skills have saved the elderly artist, stone-deaf and ailing, from the obsequies being prepared by the indistinct but menacing figures holding their own conspiracy in the background.

And who might they be? They might be priests, they might be demons.

An attachment

In a particularly harrowing moment recounted in 1943 by the diarist Friedrich Reck and taken up again by W.G. Sebald in his book *Luftkrieg und Literatur*, a woman trying to board a refugee train out of Hamburg drops her battered suitcase. Its contents spill out, and they include "toys, a manicure case, singed underwear. And last of all, the roasted corpse of a child, shrunk like a mummy, which its half-deranged mother had been carrying about with her." His translator Anthea Bell comments that any woman, and especially a mother, understands this as a natural action.

Her comment reminds me of a story told to me by a general practitioner whose patient eventually confessed to him that she had kept her papyraceous stillborn child in a cardboard box at the back of her dressing cabinet for twenty years. The mother never told the surviving child about the parchment twin who had died in the womb. She couldn't bring herself to part from her *other* child.

Collectivist and solipsist

Rationality in the old Britain was co-extensive with what humans did; it was practice-dependent: this is the view of the later Wittgenstein.

The Enlightenment conception of rationality is that it transcends all practices and cultures: this is the view of the young Wittgenstein.

Rabelais at large

When I practised as a doctor in Strasbourg, I used to cut out articles about the local dialect from a medical quarterly, *Alsamed*, and stick them in my scrapbook. This series of inserts, by far the most interesting items in the journal, managed over a couple of years to cover all the major body systems and common symptoms by providing, in three adjoining columns, the French, German and the

Elsaesserditsch (Alsatian) dialect term. Alcoholic cardiomyopathy, for instance, was entered as "lipomatose cardiaque" and "Fettherz", followed by a long list of the native terms for what was a relatively common condition in one of the major beer and wine producing regions of Europe. "E Schilkemer Bierherz" was the name given to the condition suffered by the employees of the various breweries in and around Schiltigheim. And since most of the wine drunk in Strasbourg until the early twentieth-century came from the Wolxheim region near Molsheim, the problem was also known as a "Wolxemer Winherz".

What struck me about these articles was the combative bluntness of Elsaesserditsch, and its relish for what is called the vulgar body. Organ systems such as the lung, eyes and even the heart were relatively poorly endowed with descriptive terms, but in respect of the gastrointestinal system and the urinary apparatus, the dialect came into its own. "Er het Blumekehl am Kellerfenschter"—he's got cauliflowers growing on the cellar window, for an unfortunate suffering from multiple haemorrhoids. The urologist is vulgarly known as "de Pissforscher" or "de Sprenzkannemekaniker" (watering-can fixer). There are almost a hundred Alsatian terms for the penis, some of them quite droll: "de dritt Fues" (third foot), "de Husschschlissel" (house key) or more poetically "de Paradiesschlissel" (key to paradise); and in a different register "de Musikanteknoche" (pied piper's bone), "Spritzbein" (a kind of ejaculatory pod) or plain "d'Wurscht" (sausage). "Jätz geht's um d'Wurscht, Liabling!" as one of the characters says in the grotesque, often erotic cartoons by the local humourist and children's book author, Tomi Ungerer.

That giant of European literature, Gargantua, had urological fantasies too. On a visit to Paris in chapter seventeen of Rabelais's classic First Book, he drowns the city: "[untying] his fair *Braguette*, and drawing out his *mentul* into the open aire, he so bitterly all-to-bepist them, that he drowned two hundred and sixty thousand, foure hundred and eighteen, besides the women and little children."

One of the first translations of Rabelais into another European tongue (well before Sir Thomas Urquhart's Scottish-inflected version from which I quote) was into the German of the Rhine valley, *Abenteuerliche und ungeheuerliche Geschichtsschrift vom Leben, Raten und Taten der Helden und Herren Grandgusier Gargantua und Pantagruel*. It was published in 1575 by a Strasbourg (or Strassburg, as it then was) lawyer and publicist Johann Fischart, who found the original so congenial that his version manages to be a third longer still. (Sir Thomas Urquhart's version also overran.) Fischart edits out religious or hermetic sequences, changes the characters into Rhine Valley revellers, inflates Rabelais' proverbs, epithets and ditties so as to create even more splendid word-museums and, in best Grobian fashion, lingers long over the pleasures of eating and drinking.

Milan Kundera points out in an interview that the farther east you go in Europe the greater Rabelais's influence has been: modern literature in central Europe is beholden to the late appearance of the Frenchman's writings in their national languages. A small group of Czech language specialists calling themselves "the Bohemian Thélème" translated and published *Gargantua* in 1911, with the other books following. Almost at the same time, Tadeusz Boy-Zelenski produced what is reputedly a magnificent Polish translation, one of the main influences on another of my preferred writers, the enigmatic Witold Gombrowicz.

INASMUCH

Nietzsche got it wrong: the great struggle isn't "Christ or Dionysos", but "Christ or Asclepios". That was the opposition which dominated the end of the Roman world, between the second and fifth centuries of the first millennium. Christ was exalted as a "true physician", who cured soul and body—not just in his own Passion, but also by killing off the "old Adam" in the believer's heart.

This was to be one of the tensions running through our civilisation: how to reconcile an art that sought to heal the body with a religious attitude that saw illness as a means of identification with the suffering Christ? Put yourself in God's hands, and remember the instruction: "Verily I say unto you, inasmuch as ye have done it unto one of the least of these my brethren, ye have done it unto me" (Matthew 15:40).

And remember it declines a few verses later in the negative, too.

An ultimate form of duality

It was Erasmus Darwin, grandfather of the more famous Charles, who first speculated in his 1794 treatise *Zoönomia* on the evolutionary origins of disease. In spite of the current cultural prominence of evolutionary theory, medical schools are hesitant about providing an evolutionary approach to understanding problems of human health. Like the history of medicine, it is only ever taught as an optional extra. It is indeed curious how medical practice resists any kind of *ad fontes*—a return to the beginnings. (It might simply be too embarrassing for the profession.)

Evolutionary theory provides ultimate explanations in contrast to the proximate explanations of clinical medicine, which lay out a plausible hypothesis of cause and effect, followed by a diagnosis and appropriate treatment. Ultimate explanations are (to say the least) ambitious and may sometimes have a teleological cast to them. Diabetes can be understood proximately as an impairment of insulin release in the pancreas and receptor cell sensitivity, or ultimately as a mismatch between early biology and the nutritional setting in which most humans in developed countries now find themselves. Ultimate explanations attempt to suggest how a trait or vulnerability came to exist in the first place: they may be adaptive in origin such as neoteny (retardation of mature features) or adiposity at birth (humans are the fattest neonate mammal), the latter fact being of some importance in view of our propensity to lay down adipose tissue and put on weight. They are more obviously called for in very rare cases of atavism, as the exception which proves the rule, when babies are born with tails or accessory nipples. There was also the case of the man who developed chest pain and was taken to a Texas hospital a few years ago where it was found that he had a "snake heart", in other words a single ventricle reptilian heart that was distributing mixed blood to both his systemic and pulmonary circulations. His heart also lacked the "compaction" seen in mammalian ventricles, and the coronary arteries had multiple small fistulous openings into the ventricle. (The story is a reminder that genes for primitive traits haven't disappeared; they are simply deactivated.) Some evolutionary findings can be counterintuitive: population genetic studies have shown that the ability to digest the sugars present in milk was only recently acquired by humans (approx. 10 000 years ago)—the default ancestral condition is lactose intolerance and malabsorption. The domestication of cattle and human genetic changes have gone hand in hand.

It is true to observe that evolutionary understanding of the human organism has long played a part in the prevention and management of infectious diseases: it is impossible to think of antimicrobials without considering the vast populations and short generation times that are subject to strong selection pressure from our own indiscriminate use of these useful drugs, and our own immune systems. Understanding the influenza virus is only the most visible form of evolutionary biology. Even the language used to talk about antibiotic resistance (as if it were a surprising or emergent phenomenon) hides the fact that it is readily predictable from the theory of evolution and selection pressures.

On the other hand, it is easy to understand how somebody with a true vocation to be a helper could be shocked and dismayed by the "ultimacy" of evolutionary biological explanations—there was a time when doctors were not embarrassed by mere helplessness, being obliged to offer themselves to their patients as the only really effective remedy, even in times of plague. It is even possible to imagine ultimate explanations being misused to fob off patients, as if medicine needed to be emancipated from the neediness of others—as the American poet Amy Clampitt puts it:

> that backhand, roundabout
> refusal to assume responsibility
> known as Natural Selection.

The whole point of doctors being there is to be *proximate*. Although occasionally they wilt under the slablike feeling that culture in general finds it a struggle to account for our being in the world.

A FLOWER IN THE BREASTCAGE

Botany played a central role, as the substantial part of *materia medica* and whetted by early Renaissance interest in the Greek physician and pharmacist Dioscorides, in the development of modernity, bringing together medicine and science, commerce and expanding empire, and the new scope accorded to the eye by magnification and microscopes. Dr Nicolaes Tulp, as portrayed in the famous painting, took his name from the tulip, which was then a highly speculative source of income for many Dutch businessmen, and had its image hung on a shingle outside his home and business.

TITRATING THE MIRACLE CURE

Jesus's wonder-working abilities appear to have had a dose-strength effect. The blind man from Bethesda in Mark's gospel (Mark 8:23) says to him, after his eyes are touched, "I see men, but they are like trees, walking." Full vision is restored only by a second imposition of the healing hands.

(Somewhere Aristotle writes—rather poetically—that trees are people daydreaming.)

BENEFITS OF A WHITE LIE

In her book of recollections *Meine ungeschriebenen Memoiren* (1974) Katia Mann—wife of the novelist Thomas—raises the possibility that the ill-defined health problem that afflicted her after the birth of her fourth child (she had six children altogether) and led to her Munich doctors sending her to spend months at a time in various fashionable retreats in the Swiss valleys might "have cleared up of itself" even had her wealthy parents not been able to fork out the money for the cure at Dr Friedrich Jessen's Waldsanatorium in Davos. Four years before she published her memoir, a lung specialist, Professor Christian Virchow, had looked at the well-preserved X-ray films from 1912 and told her that for all his "intensive study there was no finding to suggest incipient tuberculosis."

Katia Mann, according to Inge and Walter Jens in their biography *Frau Thomas Mann* (2003), wasn't prepared to countenance any talk of a diagnostic error—"meaning of course that *The Magic Mountain* novel would in significant parts have been based on a medical mistake." Error or not, it wouldn't detract in the least from the novel, which at one level explores all the possibilities of wilfulness and perversity, and not always those generated by what we term "illnesses." German doctors don't contradict their rich patients who have private insurance today, quite the reverse; and there is no reason to imagine they did so in the 1910s either. This practice has been called "opulence-based medicine."

Katia Mann died in 1980, aged 97.

Emetics

In 1695, the great German philosopher Wilhelm von Leibniz wrote a treatise (*De novo antidysenterico americano*) on ipecacuanha, the dried root of a plant whose name was derived from the Tupi language ("roadside sick-making plant") and first imported into Europe from Brazil by the Dutch physician Wilhelm Piso in 1641. It became a fashionable treatment after it was introduced to Paris by the physician Adrien Helvétius, who used it to relieve Louis XIV of his griping pains during one of his frequent bouts of distemper. It was in fact still available until very recently as "syrup of ipecac": every emergency room had a bottle of it in a cupboard somewhere.

Leibniz was less interested in using the syrup as an iatrochemical purgative for the ejection of "corrupt elements" than in the experimental use of emetics in order to observe what was going on in the stomach where aggregate matter was thought to be transformed into the vital substances that kept the corporeal entity alive. Digestion was almost a metaphysical category, and emesis—like autopsy—provided a forced record of what was ordinarily hidden inside.

Besides writing in fulsome terms about ipecac, Leibniz used his treatise to make proposals for the reorganisation of medicine as an institution, recommending such things as proper record keeping. He even drew a daring parallel between ancient divinatory practices and almanacs and the compilation of health data for entire populations: "the Bills of mortality of London, from which able men have drawn conclusions of consequence."

The following year, annoyed that nobody had followed up his call to make medicine more philosophical or to reorganise it along the lines of religious orders, he wrote to Guillaume François de l'Hospital: "May it please God that it should come about that doctors philosophise, and philosophers occupy themselves with medicine ['que les philosophes medicinassent']."

Among the Methodists

Booked into a hotel called The Wesley (which proclaimed itself "the first ethical hotel") near Euston Station in order to attend a conference on the boundaries of illness, I gave a thought to Methodism and its founder. Wesley's magnum opus was his book *The Doctrine of Original Sin* (1757), written at a time when more optimistic views of human nature were beginning to break through the doctrine which, for centuries, had dominated the political and personal thinking of Christian Europe. When Wesley wrote his tract, inveighing against his own generation and its belief in the "dignity of human nature", even churchmen were loath to acknowledge the full weight of the original doctrine. As Wesley saw, if human nature was in "perfect health", then why did Protestant rationalism have need of "Christian philosophy" which was "the only true method of healing a distempered soul"? He was quoting Plato, but pagan words were good enough. Wesley's chief item of evidence was *Gulliver's Travels*, in which Jonathan Swift similarly lambasted human self-love and spiritual pride. Wesley sought to remind modern rationalists of the old anxieties in order to make it clear that "unregenerate" human beings—lumped with deformities and "dead in sin"—would always be in need of religious therapy: in so doing, he was also universalising the concept of illness, a recalibration of human priorities we are better placed to appreciate than he was.

OMNIPRATICIEN

"Il faut être spécialiste de tout," wrote the jazz trumpeter and literary provocateur Boris Vian, at the beginning of what the French call *les trente glorieuses*—the thirty fat years after the war that made them wealthy as never before.

After 1968, if you weren't a specialist you were, for the ordinary citizen, infra dig. "Mais vous n'êtes que généraliste…" How many times I had to absorb the implied humiliation, chatting to the locals who came into my practice in the rue Wimpheling in the northern district of Strasbourg out of sheer curiosity.

Well, not that many times, if the truth be told. That's why I'm not there anymore.

LUNGS AND LAUGHTER

There is a kind of laughter "that has no lungs behind it," according to Franz Kafka. That is precisely the kind of stifled amusement I heard as a student doing the rounds in the chest wards of the Royal Infirmary in Glasgow. Patients with bronchiectasis coughing up buckets of sputum flecked with blood and pus every morning, and somehow still finding reasons to be cheerful.

In his cultural history of the body, *Anatomies*, Hugh Aldersley-Williams fails even to mention the lungs—those "proud strong tormented imperturbable creatures", as Kafka imagined them.

Katherine Mansfield—a consumptive like Kafka—thought of her lungs as birds, which may explain why so many of her stories are about creatures which seek to fly. She suffered a fatal pulmonary haemorrhage running up the stairs to show Middleton Murry how well she was.

THE ELECT PLACE

Thomas de Quincey lay troubled in his opium dreams by the oceanic apparitions of human faces—"faces upturned to the heavens: faces, imploring, wrathful, despairing, surged upwards by thousands, by myriads, by generations, by centuries." They tyrannised his sleep. He hadn't thought that death could undo so many, and the spectacle horrified him. His disquiet brought to mind the epitaph the historian Fernand Braudel quotes from the writings of Pollard and Crossley, historians of the Industrial Revolution, that "two generations were sacrificed to the creation of an industrial base" in the United Kingdom—"sent like fuel to feed the factory-smoke," in Ruskin's terrible phrase (*The Nature of Gothic*).

Humphrey Carpenter's haunting mosaic-anthology *Pandaemonium: The Coming of the Machine as Seen by Contemporary Observers* (1985) contains exhilarated descriptions of the industrial country that Britain was becoming, such as Fanny Kemble's awed description of the "beautiful road to Hades" constructed by Brunel beneath the Thames, and the very first descriptions of Stevenson's railway between Manchester and Liverpool. They sit cheek by jowl with a desolate and helpless awareness of the blighted countryside, polluted towns and stunted working people—the price paid by a small country for its global supremacy in manufacturing and trade.

Already by Blake's time, the British Isles had gone through several cycles of dispossession of the peasantry and the growth of agricultural innovation and market competition. Without the removal of the means of subsistence at the most basic level it would not have been possible to introduce the wage relations that were such a striking feature of British life at a time when most of the European continent was still feudal. Dispossessed families were moving into the towns while Calvinist theology made it possible for their masters to assuage any lingering guilt about the fate of their fellow men and women and reap their own landed fortune. When Blake wrote in *Jerusalem* "all things begin and end in Albion's ancient ruined Druid rocky shore," it was not so much the sceptred isle of socio-political stability he had in mind as the island of despoliations and desolations, events which it resists, absorbs, and finally exports to the world. Uprooted people, according to Simone Weil, either fall into a death-like lethargy or expend their energy in some activity "necessarily designed to uproot, often by the most violent methods, those who are not yet uprooted, or only partly so." Modernity in lowland Britain scarred the landscape in a way that is hardly apparent on the continent, where the French, for instance, are able to have their weekly markets and run high-speed trains, and the Germans, for all that their cities were bombed out of recognition in the mid-twentieth century, can still boast thriving and distinct regional cultures.

This was the island—with its scenes of misery and degradation, its middens and dank alleys and cinder-heaps—that grieved Ruskin so greatly. "Beauty has been in the world since the world was made, and human language can make a shift, somehow, to give account of it, whereas the peculiar forces of devastation induced by modern city life have only entered the world lately; and no existing terms of language known to me are enough to describe the forms of filth, and modes of ruin, that varied themselves along the course of Croxted Lane." (*Fiction, Fair and Foul*).

Something of De Quincey's drugged imaginings turn up in Saul Bellow's celebrated sentence in *Seize the Day*: "And the great crowd, the inexhaustible current of millions of every race and kind pouring out, pressing round, of every age, of every genius, possessors of every human secret, antique and future, in every face the refinement of one particular motive or essence—I *labor*, I *spend*, I *strive*, I *design*, I *love*, I *cling*, I *uphold*, I *give away*, I *envy*, I *long*, I *die*, I *hide*, I *want*."

Both writers surely had in mind Dante's icy lines about the "mille visi" of *Inferno* 32:

> Then I saw a thousand faces there,
> Blue with the cold; it makes me shudder
> And always will, when I think of those frozen shallows.

Empty masks

The dissidence of the student movement in the 1960s has spread to nearly every sphere of life. Everyone's subjectivity is allowed a moral and conceptual bolthole, with full consumer rights added, but there is nothing especially subversive about this turning away from the objective order: on the contrary, it is apolitical, inward and quietist. The 1972 manifesto of the Heidelberg Socialist Patients' Collective, "Turn Illness into a Weapon", attempted to make revolutionary subjects out of the feeling of sickness (real or imagined) generated by a society in which utility maximisation and economic optimisation defined what was rational. Pathos and abjection were somehow going to liberate the said subjects from the ravages of "iatrocapitalism".

One reason for this turning away may be because we have all been inoculated, culturally at least, with a dose of Vedic disbelief in the self, of "non-ego theory". We want to shed our idiocy, in the original sense of the word.

Sound and image

A short silent black-and-white film shows the ailing Sigmund Freud on the terrace of his new house at 20 Maresfield Gardens after his family's emigration to London in the wake of the Nazi annexation of Austria in 1938. Freud refused to be filmed and recorded at the same time, in other words to have his physical representation augmented by his vocal traits, or his expressive voice to be given solidity by his bodily movements: he did not want to allow a memorialisation in image *and* sound to insinuate that his essence had somehow been caught. The distinguished old iconoclast had clearly anticipated that the body-mind split would play itself out in a later era as an anxiety about image and reality.

Beautiful Souls

Like the kibbutzim, post-war British society was virtuous, quite knowingly and sometimes smugly so. It was virtuous in the way that Americans implant innocence in their children; it was part of an only partly explicit programme of social engineering. And the beautiful souls of this virtuous society were the doctors.

At least the British refused to play the game of prisoner's dilemma as if it were a rule for society in general rather than a calculated and strategic move in the Cold War. But it was the advocacy of game theory—ironically by the trendiest of counter-culture people like R. D. Laing—that finally did for the communitarian spirit of the United Kingdom once the Thatcher years got under way.

A figure like the GP was only possible under the benevolent oversight of social liberalism: market liberalism—a quite different creed—was bound to undermine the established ways of the "better classes" and the patrician assumptions of "those who know best." Wanting to help others became slightly suspect. Students no longer had vocations. As John Gray puts it, "perhaps the most salient feature of our age is not a decline in individual liberty but the vanishing of authority, and a concomitant metamorphosis of moral judgements into a species of personal preferences, between which reason is powerless to arbitrate."

What is the Value of a Profession?

Nietzsche knew the exact value of a profession. "A profession makes us thoughtless: therein lies its greatest blessing. For it is a bulwark, behind which we are allowed to withdraw when qualms and worries of a general kind attack us." In the old days it was possible to suggest that if you knew what a person did, then almost everything about him had already been said.

That era of self-confident thoughtlessness has passed; medicine is anthropologically strange to those who practise it. And doctors suspect that reality is now articulated in another idiom, the idiom of that sacrificial system called the market that has helped to defer violence and keep the peace in Europe for fifty years. An advanced industrial society no longer requires rationality from its consumers; only its producers are required to maintain it, and for reasons of safety and efficiency their working methods have to resemble those of the airline industry as closely as possible.

Only thus is it possible to understand the enthusiasm for checklists in Atul Gawande's anodyne book *The Checklist Manifesto: How to Get Things Right*. Checklists against errors of ignorance and ineptitude might make perfect sense on the technical side of medicine but the closer you get to people assailed by qualms and worries of a general kind the less appropriate they become. Some degree of ignorance and ineptitude might even be necessary qualities for a good doctor. Doctors used to know how to deal with mortal fright and distress, because they were often helpless themselves.

A SPINOZISM

The critic Walter Benjamin remarks that in his famous novel Proust's narrator was able to weep on the death of his grandmother only when he bent down to take his shoes off on the evening of the event. His bending down, Benjamin suggests, was the means to his expression of grief. "In this way, the body is what rouses a profound pain; and it can serve no less to arouse profound thought." Benjamin was ahead of his time, insofar as it is now recognised that affective conditions are intimately related to body postures.

It is perhaps curious then that the psychologists who came up with the famous 7-38-55 rule (the respective percentages for verbal component, voice tone and facial expression in the communication of affect) did not think posture had a role to play in conveying the emotions. Such is the prestige of the face, as Emmanuel Levinas insists in his philosophy.

Another kind of nosology

Allopathic medicine turns on metonymy, the notion that disturbances in bodily function can be ascribed to the functioning of individual organs, which then become the domain of expertise for various specialists; diagnoses in traditional Chinese medicine (and many other alternative therapies) work on a metaphoric basis. The western ability to separate emotions and physical functions has much to do with this dichotomy; although Chinese medicine talks about the abnormalities of an organ system—especially of the heart, liver and kidney—these diagnoses are not to be understood as referring to actual physical disease processes affecting that organ, but to *metaphors* for what in the West would be regarded as emotional dispositions. An emotion in the Western sense expresses itself through somatic signs and symptoms which can be read by an experienced Chinese practitioner. In the traditional nosology, "liver" is a metaphor for anger, "heart" for anxiety, "spleen" for melancholy and "kidney" for reproductive potency. Not to treat an angry liver might lead to it attacking the spleen, i.e. repressed rage expressing itself as depression. Catharsis is an alien meaning in this context; what counts is re-establishing the original harmony of the organs.

A ritual humbling

We have become so besotted with the new pieties of the school of solicitude that we forget that becoming a patient means to be a person stripped of pride.

Therapeutic subjectivism

Perhaps the whole attractiveness of remedies conceived on the homeopathic model is that they produce not so much a resolution of the disease (which, on the allopathic model, is an external aggressor) as a reconciliation of the person with his constitution. The disease is *cajoled* to bring forth the cure from within itself.

The hollow of a body

Delacroix summed up human life in his early painting *Le lit défait*, which can be seen at the museum in his old house in the rue Furstenberg in Paris. Unlike Tracey Emin's vapid exhibition piece "My bed", which is just a mess, with the unmade bed and its environs strewn with empty bottles of booze, fag-ends, newspapers, uneaten tidbits and used condoms—"revealing she's as insecure and imperfect as the rest of the world" according to the official Saatchi Gallery site—Delacroix's watercolour shows the absence of the human presence in a scene that bears its very imprint.

This bed is still warm. Where folds and drapes had been important in earlier art as indicating nobility, here the roiled linen constitutes the most banal scene, being the apparently haphazard surface features of a bed in a room empty even of furniture. Yet these innocent white cotton folds, just under the distressed pillow, conceal a Medusa's head (once seen not forgotten, like an army recruitment poster); and somebody else has suggested there may be a flayed head at the foot of the bed (though I have yet to identify it and hope not to find it).

The hidden drama of Delacroix's seemingly benign palimpsest of a bed without an occupying human presence verges on the artistic movement that would later be known as Expressionism. And come to think of it: billowing linen and laundry would return as popular themes for the Impressionists too.

Psychobabble

The depressed woman in the late David Forster Wallace's story "The Depressed Person" (in *Brief Interviews with Hideous Men*) is stuck in the inward drift of her own ego, speaking a ghastly idiom absorbed from TV shows, million-selling inevitable MD-authored self-help books and the general ambience. It is a shock to pick up Dante's great poem and realise that Hell is precisely the babble of those locked inside their own minds. And how did the depressed woman get there other than through the usual good intentions of those who always want to make Hell a better place?

One point: she must have had a good health insurance policy to get a psychiatrist who would want to *listen* to her, and not just rush her out of the door with a prescription for psychoactive medication. To sign a prescription line for medications is three times more lucrative in terms of doctor-hours than the talking cure.

"Postmen like doctors"

In his memoir *A Sense of Place*, the historian Richard Cobb recalls his favourite uncle, a country doctor who often took him along on rounds: "He was a tremendous gossip, and endlessly inquisitive about people; indeed, I think he only practised medicine in order to get into other people's houses. I would sit waiting in the car while he did the rounds, and, after each visit, he would come to the car triumphantly with some new item of malice, rather like a researcher after a good day in the Archives Nationales." This love of a chosen past and small-scale scenery fed into Cobb's distrust of methodology (which carried him all the way through a career as a distinguished historian of modern France): "Why do historians spend so much time arguing, imposing definitions, proposing 'models', when they could be getting on with their research?" He thought there was nothing more boring than abstract speculation about what history *is*—you just did it, and didn't spare a further thought for its social function. He liked to begin his investigations with a specific person in a time and place. His model was Inspector Maigret—"a historian of habit, of the déjà vu… a historian of the unpredictable… a historian of class", who is unceasingly alert to "habit, routine, assumption, banality, everydayness, seasonability, popular conservatism." Richard Cobb was, in short, more of a novelist than a conventional historian.

This desire to read other people's letters, to enter the inner sanctum of other people's homes, to open a door on their lives stayed with Cobb all *his* life: it is what he claims "being, or becoming, a historian is all about." This compulsion—a young man home from university following his country-doctor relative on his rounds—also drives the first part of Thomas Bernhard's novel *Verstörung* (translated as *Gargoyles*), although in its historical context the "malice" which all so often surfaces in the Austrian rural setting has a nightmarish aspect to it too. "It would be wrong to refuse to face the fact," the father counsels his rationalist son, "that everything is *fundamentally sick and sad*."

That is not at all the conclusion reached by Cobb, who in later life became a nostalgist for Paris before it became the wealthy capital city of the *trente glorieuses*. He did however retain a liking for the odd, the marginal, and the unclassifiable. And his writings suggest that the historian's task is even weightier than the doctor's—as well as being one which offers moments of levity and true radiance. The historian has to truffle through the records for the untold anecdote, for what has eluded memory and recollection, and perhaps lain unnoticed for years in some yellowing dossier. He has (if he is worth his title of historian) to treat all testimony like a disbeliever. Then he sentences people to life—in all its saltiness and strangeness.

LITERATURE AND MEDICINE

To refer to a writer as a *medical* writer is to place him or her into a more distinct and indulgent category that softens the reader up for something less than the real thing, and insinuates that any falling short in terms of literary style will be made up for by a dose of honest-to-God authenticity.

AN OBIT

"Ultimately he was overwhelmed by his own exacting standards and took his own life." The regret of this very Henry Jamesian phrase stood out among the usually anodyne obituary notices for doctors in the *British Medical Journal*. I wondered how many and what kind of sufferings had been compacted into that opening adverb.

THE NEW CONFLICT OF THE FACULTIES

What makes for a good doctor? Thick books have been written on this question, and it has been worried over in ethics courses, learned articles and parliamentary select committees: the *British Medical Journal* once had a theme issue breezily titled "What's a good doctor, and how can you make one?" The question is still open, because its logic is flawed. Why should good people be *made*? Perhaps the whole issue becomes easier to grasp if we look first at an allied profession, and ask a slightly differently phrased question. What makes for a good lawyer, we might ask, specifically a good criminal lawyer?

The ambiguous standing of the legal profession—and it is surely a point that helps to topple the advocate Clamence from his pedestal in Camus' *La Chute* (1956)—is that "a good lawyer" is a term of aesthetic approval rather than one of ethical appraisal. A good barrister or advocate is an effective orator, a manipulator of language and argument, a performer who plays the part. Whether justice is seen to be done is not of primary concern for the lawyer, though it may well be for his or her client. American court-room dramas tell us repeatedly that nothing swells a lawyer's reputation as much as winning cases, especially those thought by fellow lawyers to be difficult or even indefensible (if the plaintiff is indeed guilty as charged). A good lawyer is someone who wins cases.

The moral dilemma is outlined succinctly by the hero of *Catcher in the Rye*: "Even if you *did* go around saving guys' lives, and all, how would you know if you did it because you really *wanted* to save guys' lives, or because what you *really* wanted to do was be a terrific lawyer, with everybody slapping you on the back and congratulating you in court when the goddam trial was over... How would you know you weren't being a phony? The trouble is, you *wouldn't*." Camus' lawyer has a further problem of moral perspective: he wants to be a judge, a judge who appeals above the heads of those in the fictional court to the wider court of public opinion. The rulings of judges are, of course, generally treated as an absolute declaration of what is right and true. Those sinister, impossibly distant figures in Kafka come to mind, or the elevated figure of the Lord High Chancellor superintending the Court of the Chancery in Dickens' *Bleak House*, with "foggy glory round his head."

Clamence mistakes the closed world of the Law, which is essentially a serious kind of game, for the larger world in which clients suffer. His "fall" is to experience that suffering himself.

It is a nice paradox that lawyers owe their status in society and their income to a form of injustice: if the law were respected by all, as Karl Marx and many others have gleefully pointed out, there would be no lawyers. There would be no need for them. Crimes and misdemeanours keep lawyers in business. In would hardly be in the interests of the criminal justice system to repress crime to the point at which lawyers go out of business—and make no mistake, a thousand lawyers with no clients would be a far worse prospect for society than a thousand petty criminals on the loose: just look at the French Revolution. No lawyer is therefore entitled to believe, like Clamence, in his fundamental innocence.

It is noteworthy that lawyers as a profession were abhorrent to the sectarians of the English Civil War. "He eats up all that comes within his power; for this Proverb is true, goe to Law, and none shall get but the Lawyer. The Law is the Fox, poore men are the geesse; he pulls of their feathers, and feeds upon them," wrote Gerrard Winstanley, in his famous tract *Fire in the Bush* (1650). Puritans disliked lawyers for the same reason that they objected to the theatre: what they put on was a sham, a hypocrisy, a sensuous spectacle that could distract the sinner from the contemplation of God and his need for redemption. They didn't like people who put it on. Nothing in public life was worse than the masquerade of imposture, of people giving airs and pretending to be what they weren't. Christian, the main character of John Bunyan's *Pilgrim's Progress* is misdirected by Mr Worldly-Wiseman to seek counsel of Mr. Legality, "a cheat" who dwells in the village of Morality. Mr Legality was skilled, no doubt, in circumvention of the laws.

What about good doctors? Here, the issue is at first sight not so clouded. Doctors derive their income too, from a kind of evil—from those natural evils, disease and illness. These are not chosen or desired in the same way that the Law is dishonoured intentionally, by an act of will. By the middle of the twentieth century, medicine had acquired the art of true healing, and was able to distance itself to a large extent, if not entirely from the kind of professional masquerade and theatricality which Pascal objected to: "Reason never wholly overcomes imagination, while the contrary is quite common… If physicians did not have long gowns and mules, if learned doctors did not wear square caps and robes four sizes too large, they would never have deceived the world, which finds such an authentic display irresistible. If they possessed true justice, and if physicians possessed the true art of healing, they would not need square caps; the majesty of such sciences would command respect in itself. But, as they only possess imaginary science, they have to resort to these vain devices in order to strike the imagination, which is their real concern, and this, in fact, is how they win respect."

Increasingly, however, medicine operates in the field of choice. Instead of the descriptive laws of science and observed patterns of conformity—laws *of*—medical practice is dominated by the prescriptive laws of probabilistic reasoning—laws *for*. Much of the workload of an ordinary doctor includes screening for risk factors and providing advice about aspects of ordinary life which have been colonised by the goddess Fortuna, that is by choice and possibility: birth control is an obvious instance. That is why some people object to the use of the word "patient" to describe the person who seeks advice. Think too of preventive medicine with its "numbers needed to treat" and the impossibility to explaining risk to the ordinary patient. (It is a considerable handicap for its rational gospel that most doctors do not understand probabilistic thinking either, as the German psychologist Gert Gigerenzer has shown in several embarrassing papers.) But then the entire universe of risk management is predicated on your being a case within a mass abstraction, not a flesh-and-blood person.

In short, medicine has become less innocent, more like the law. It has shifted into the territory not of logic but of rhetoric. The implicit contract between a doctor and an ill person seems to have taken on all kinds of extraneous baggage, even the client status that pertains in the legal setting. Does legal address have an equivalent in medicine though?

Herman Melville's *The Confidence Man* shows us how the salesman parodies the preacher. So what about the doctor, all too knowingly aware that he is a drug? Should he "sell" his doctrine, when medicine can't save? Well, in fact he's in the business of selling hope, which always seems to involve the term "might help". Hope is, of course, pure crack, utterly addictive, the ultimate stuff. In his lowly social position, the priest represents a power that is greater than himself, and although this power is not his own, he becomes, by dint of it, a power himself. Whose representative is the doctor? As the elderly Count Shabelsky remarks to the pompous young doctor in Chekhov's play *Ivanov*: "Doctors are like lawyers, only lawyers just rob you, while doctors rob and murder you to boot. Present company excepted."

Pense-bête, guide-âne

French idioms for "checklist" leave no doubt that such bureaucratically inspired mnemonic devices are not held in great esteem in the culture that prides itself most on thinking explicitly (and often at great length) about why we do what we do—and honours its thinkers commensurately.

Sthenia

A few years ago, I enjoyed an epistolary discussion with a distinguished colleague about the term "asthenia", which I used to hear from some of my French patients (who came to me complaining of "asthénie"). He told me it can be found not only in the International Classification of Diseases (ICD9) but as a "preferred term" in the Dictionary of Adverse Reactions (MedDRA). It is therefore a unique signifier absorbing lower-level terms such as adynamia, debility, neurasthenia, loss of energy and fatigue. It is also jocularly known (to health professionals) as TATT: "tired all the time."

Asthenia turns up on every other page of Novalis's notebook *Das allgemeine Brouillon*, written on the cusp of the nineteenth century but edited and published only in the early years of the twentieth in Germany, and translated another century on into English by David W. Wood, as *Notes for a Romantic Encyclopedia* (2007).

So too does its positive form, *sthenia*, which is never seen these days at all (although that's not entirely true, now I think about it: I saw it once, in a French psychiatric report I translated, about a patient who developed paranoid delusions after taking corticosteroids). "Sthenia" was coined by the Scottish physician John Brown (1735–88), a favourite of the eminent William Cullen (known to his students at Edinburgh University as "Old Spasm"). Brown was by all accounts an ambitious if eccentric physician who aspired in his *Elementa Medicinae* (1780) to find a universal principle that would account for all medical phenomena: every human is born with a certain quotient of irritability or excitability. Deficient excitation engenders asthenia, excess sthenia. Excitability, for some physicians in the eighteenth century, was the source of vitality. "Life is a forced state."

Although Novalis never read Brown's texts, he certainly picked up on the new psychoperceptual scheme through his discussions with friends about Schelling's *Von der Welt-Seele* and other contemporary and speculative works of natural philosophy. For a speculative thinker in search of a unified or universal science, Brown's theory must have had some appeal. It allowed him to incorporate older humeral notions and Paracelsian notions of "chemistry". Novalis does however express some dissatisfaction with Brown's Newtonian ambitions at one point ("Brown has completely failed to explain disease"), and at another he says: "Irritability is increased by abstraction. Too much abstraction produces asthenia—too much reflection, sthenia. I must reflect a lot more and abstract a lot less. I already possess enough irritability.

An acute thinker is a *sensitive* meter—an extremely subtle reagent." (297) "Abstractions" must be those externally imposed structures that Blake identified as other men's systems; "reflections" are self-generated.

Liddell and Scott's Greek dictionary tells us that "sthenia" was customarily used as an epithet for Zeus—"the powerful." It would be the rare patient who enters the medical surgery and booms across the table at his doctor: "I feel like Zeus today—what are you going to do about it, man?" (Or admits, like the apostle Paul, that all his dynamism or power accomplishes itself in weakness.) 2 Cor. 12:9)

Novalis's economy of health might be outdated, and some of his speculations feel like the imaginings of a literary hypochondriac, but he correctly surmises that modern medicine is more about lack than excess. "There is a deficiency in every true illness—and this gives rise to the reluctance of every illness. It is for this reason that one also says—"What is *wrong* with you?" ("Was *fehlt* dir?")

CONSUMPTION AND CONSUMMATION

You only have to watch a baby as it teases and plays with its mother's nipple after hunger has been stilled—breaking off from sucking to smile or look around at its father, lifting an unsteady hand to caress the breast, and plunging back to savour the lacteal source, perhaps this time with a playful toothless bite to the teat—to realise that the principle of deferred gratification is being already absorbed at the infant stage. An extremely complex organisation of the muscles of expression has made this blossom of a smile possible—"the first sign of the superfluous need to communicate for something other than the appeasement of a thirst", as Paul Valéry commented. Later in life, children are told not to play with their food, like the hapless children in the classic German children's book *Struwwelpeter*, and yet playing with food is the elementary social experience. It may well be that true civility presupposes not taking the straight road to our needs.

And incidentally, the only sound an infant can utter with its mouth full and its throat busily swallowing its mother's breast milk is a nasal one: a long hum of appreciation. This liquid stuff is simply too wonderful for words. Hence, as Steven Connor speculates in *Beyond Words*, the bilabial nasal sound which identifies the mother in most (if not all) languages: mmm!

This is a short-lived stage we may be more nostalgic about than we realise. The American psychologist Erik Erikson, who wrote about social trust, also pointed out in his book *Childhood and Society* that the unavoidable experience of teething—which mostly occurs after weaning—is a kind of banishment from paradise ("the ontogenetic contribution to the biblical saga of paradise"). As the teeth erupt, pain enters the infant's world: the same mouth that provided lacteal pleasure is now the source of the metaphysical wound at the heart of the universe. We learn to stop presuming this is the best of all possible worlds.

Lovin' in my baby's eyes/spectroscopy

Certain artists—above all, Rembrandt, in some of his chiaroscuro self-portraits looming out of the dark (I'm thinking of the fine example in the National Gallery of Scotland)—have the ability to shock us into recalling that the eyes, these paired membranes tremulously alive in the cluster of what seem at times to be the bizarrely protuberant features of the human face, notably the nose and ears, about which the Russian critic Mikhail Bakhtin wrote so well, are actually vulnerably jellied extrusions of cerebral tissue. Eyes are the centre of our emotions and awareness. The teenage German philosopher Novalis was so swayed by the evidence of things seen that he noted: "All our senses should become eyes." In the eyes perception reveals itself, which is why the ancient Greeks thought they could know the nature of their *daimon*, their personal fate, by looking at the pupil of another person's eyes. Walt Whitman seems to have felt this force when he commented in Brooklyn newspaper in 1846 about the novelty of a gallery display of photographic images: "For the strange fascination of looking at the eyes of a portrait, sometimes goes beyond what comes from the real orbs themselves."

These externalisations of cerebral tissue—as the great Spanish anatomist Santiago Ramón y Cajal first hypothesised—are so central to our perception of other persons' faces that we attribute spiritual qualities to their movement and colour, even though the haphazardly flecked, minutely contracting, reactive sphincter of the iris stroma—with fractal variations of blue, grey, green and hazel in the pigment frill, radial furrows and crypts—may even have something unnervingly galactic about it, especially when viewed up close. Diamonds and rust, as the song goes. Or "terrible crystal", as G. K. Chesterton referred to the eyes in a poem, "more incredible/ Than all the things they see."

Our eyes are open, wide open, yet they don't see the radiant quasar world as it is, objectively speaking—emanations older than sight itself. All we trichromatous beings can see is "visible light" at between 7000 and 4000 ångström, a tiny band of the electromagnetic spectrum that emerged from the decoupling of matter and radiation following the Big Bang. If we could see other parts of the spectrum the world would look quite different. That is why philosophy teaches people to see, but not with the lens of the eye—even if some philosophers claim to be able to peer right through that aperture and deep into the godhead.

"When a man loves a woman whose life is constantly before him," wrote Martin Buber in *Ich und Du* (*I and Thou*), in 1923, "the You that he sees shining in her eyes allows him to glimpse a ray of the eternal You." Even at the risk of worshipping an image the lover experiences a godly presence ("the eternal You") in his lover's eyes along with a dizzying awareness that even the divine ("God as love") is vulnerable.

Mind you, if eyes are all that we can read, as Voltaire suggested, then we haven't learned to read very much at all. It probably won't be the faces looming out of the dark that will come to haunt us then but the biometrics of transparency. Rembrandt used to tell people not to get too close to his paintings. Some of the paints were poisonous.

How to die

After Immanuel Kant, ethics talks uninterruptedly about the individual person assuming his or her majority in a society of the like-minded, and Ruskin writes in *Unto This Last* "for, truly, the man who does not know when to die, does not know how to live"; in practice, however, all the weight of morality has shifted from the patient to the professional, who now has to be a paragon of the virtues, unsullied by despair, imperturbable. This is most obvious in the forgotten tradition of the *ars moriendi*. Even talking about the *moriens* now seems in bad taste. We "palliate", "enhance" end-of-life care, talk about the evil of suffering (though that can't quite be what we mean), and generally do everything to draw death of what used to be called its *sting*. Pick up a diary from two hundred years ago, and it will become apparent that our ancestors worked on themselves in order to die as moral beings, in the sense that Kant would recognise in his writings on autonomy. Some even died with the book of instruction propped up in front of them.

There was even a time when Job—that "brother of jackals" and "companion of owls"—was the exemplary patient.

Circumlocutions

Empowering is surely the cant word of the millennium (along with her sister *ownership*). "Corsets are back in fashion. Not only are they eye-catching, they're empowering to wear." A less pretentious copywriter might just have said "fun to wear", but presumably it doesn't have the requisite domina ring.

The example is trivial, but it's quite common to hear people use the words they hear (prestigious) other people using: village people all over the world are being "empowered" by humanitarian groups and NGO workers. I heard someone resort to workshop jargon only a few years ago as dusk fell in a small village in Andhra Pradesh. There she stood, the embarrassed beneficiary, holding her stake. Power is surely something people acquire for themselves or it can't mean very much; having it handed to them suggests it has something in common with pity.

Elizabeth Pisani in *The Wisdom of Whores: Bureaucrats, Brothels and the Business of AIDS* mentions a game she used to play with jaded colleagues when attending conferences at which interest groups were on the prowl for government and donor funding. The rules of the game are very simple: each colleague separately prepares a list of a dozen favourite "bullshit terms", e.g. "blue-sky thinking", "touch base", "low-hanging fruit", "gamechanger", "moving forward" and so on: the first person who can tick off all the terms and display a Bullshit Bingo full card is the winner. There is a catch though: to be able to win, you have to stay awake.

Each one of these cliché-words is a mantra, one of development's buzz-words, a reason for countless studies and reports as well as meetings in expensive hotels like the one Pisani attended with her colleagues. They are part of the bland dishonesty of our age: they are employed not just to manipulate consensus but also pull the wool over people's eyes, thereby allowing interpretative scope should the situation they were meant to engineer turn out contrary to expectations. That is why bureaucrats employ them instinctively. Managers use them because they are terrified of gainsaying the company line. Euphemisms and equivocations are aspects of the lexicon everybody draws on these days.

"If you don't know the buzz words," an NGO director is quoted in *The Economist*, "you hardly have a chance to apply for funds."

Weightlessness

It may well be that "knowledge" will become so cheap that what a doctor does will strike the other members of society as being about as interesting as a bricklayer's workday. Perhaps all a heart surgeon is doing is a glorified form of plumbing. What will happen to the doctor's symbolic authority then? Will the placebo effect disappear?

A VISION OF THE HIGHER LIFE

All of higher life can be schematised to that specialised surface of revolution called the doughnut (topologists call this a *ring torus* and embryologists the process whereby a hollow ball of cells buckles to form a cup *gastrulation*): it has two dimpled vesicles or depressions which merge allowing a hole to open up in the middle that gets longer and more extenuated as the doughnut gets bigger, so that in the end the world can be taken in through the opening at the upper pole and its spoor deposited from the lower one. The digestive tract can thus be regarded as a tunnel (with ramifications) extending in a somewhat convoluted way through the body, and thus as a *hole*; or it can be regarded as an organ-system within the body, and thus as a constituent part: this is what allows us to have specialists dealing with every aspect of the tract, from the antechamber of ingested substances (stomatologists) to the temporary holding space for ejecta (proctologists). In fact, as a constituent part, the digestive tract is the site of the *microbiome*, the ecology of symbiotic micro-organisms which share our body space and provide us with a tenth of our calorific intake, manufacture vitamins and co-factors, and protect against alien intruders. The biome weighs 1.5 kilograms on average, and harbours 10 times more bacterial cells than there are cells in our "own" bodies.

"The words of a dead man are modified in the guts of the living," wrote W. H. Auden in his memorable 1939 elegy for his recently deceased precursor William Butler Yeats—but he cannot have suspected all the implications of what was then a daringly medical metaphor for the transformations of the Word. We are portable ecologies sharing symbiotic bacteria as much as we are individuals in the moral and legal sense. And even the indivisibility of the Cartesian ego may be in question. "In the vast colony of our being," suggested the Portuguese poet Fernando Pessoa, famous for being several different poets, "there are many species of people who think and feel in different ways." (He wrote that in *The Book of Disquiet*, under the name Bernardo Soares.)

All in all, the doughnut schematisation of the human body is a very Platonic vision of things, especially when we more obviously resemble hybrid superorganisms. From the point of view of the ring torus though, when the distance to the axis of revolution declines, and it becomes a horn, spindle and finally sphere, it has *degenerated*. Leonardo thought that the person of bad habits and limited reason was a mere "sack". Such persons were straightforward conduits for receiving and ejecting food and resembled other humans only in speech and shape, "and in all else are far below the level of the beasts."

Guts

So much of our emotional life is *splanchnic*. "The Song of Songs", that most gender-bending of love poems which stands in the middle of the Hebrew (and Puritan) scriptures like a laden plum-tree, has the touching refrain: "My beloved put his hand on the door-latch and my bowels yearned for him." Ivan Illich, who made the story of the Good Samaritan the whole basis of his critique of society, reminds us that the early Bible translators were speaking literally when they talked of the "bowels of compassion": the Greek word in the New Testament for taking pity, *splagnizesthai*, makes it a gut response. Centuries later, Oliver Cromwell's appeal rings down the English language to our age of compassion fatigue—"I beseech ye, in the bowels of Christ, think it possible that ye may be mistaken." His was the introduction to a truly visceral politics. Bowlahoola was Blake's digestive tract, a place of anvils and hammers and furnaces in the world's bowels where unborn souls received bodies. And let us not forget that bowels were the seat of corruption that burst out of quartered bodies, those of the still living condemned, for exhibition to the public.

The bowels are wormlike. Laid out for inspection on surgical drapes they glisten, and writhe slowly to a peristaltic time of their own, coilings and loops of the serpent from the Garden of Eden—and some Gnostic sources even suggest that God incorporated the snake as the digestive tract of his two proto-humans after that notorious incident with the fruit of the Tree of Knowledge. The viscera, according to the Montpellier school, were believed to have relative autonomy and independent sensibility. They were part of the unconscious, the *vegetative* life, a notion which was current well before Freud. For evolutionary theorists, guts are probably what made the difference during the so-called Cambrian Explosion when the world's zoology shifted from being dominated by bacteria, algae and plankton to the complexity of multicellular animals.

Nowadays, in the world of the spectacle, Americans (and the rest of us who aspire to be Americans) spill theirs on talk shows, and figurative guts still don't seem any easier to cram back in again, even for shrinks.

Proactive patients

The market has made it intolerable that patients (from "patior", *to suffer or bear*) should be rendered spectators to their own needs, obliged to assume a position that advertises the unequal nature of the relationship between titled health care provider (aka "doctor", from "docere", *to teach*) and anonymous recipient.

I recall a nugatory discussion between Julia Neuberger and Raymond Tallis in the *British Medical Journal* in 1999, in a decade when the journal took on Orwellian traits in its desire to restyle medicine: Neuberger wished to do away with the word, which for her was all too redolent of passivity and suffering; some advocates, tongue in cheek, have even suggested using the acronym TIFKAP: the individual formerly known as a patient. What neither party pointed out (or seemed aware of) was that what should be a transaction between two subjects who share responsibility for the outcome had been elided into the unequal relationship between an oppressor and a victim: only victims in our society have a right to decry their status with unfeigned indignation. A person deprived of agency cannot be blamed for what is done to him.

Tallis pointed out that even in the United States, where consumerist medicine sets the tone and patients are anything but submissive, the term "patient" remains unchallenged. Neuberger looked forward to the confident service user, "informed and participative", and displayed a vision of health-care that made it seem as if health was only ever a question of lifestyle choices.

Tallis observed that words acquire new meanings through custom and usage, and that there is simply no other current word which could be used in its place.

After all, how much autonomy does a seriously ill person really enjoy, or want? She is probably quite willing to cast her welfare on the mercy of strangers. At the heart of medicine is a compassionate bond that relies on trust and acknowledges vulnerability. Tallis's final comment: "compassion may stink of paternalism (or maternalism), but without them medicine stinks."

Man-midwife

Since 1982, pursuant to a European Community resolution, it has been possible for men to practise midwifery. Very few have felt called to the profession: Italy with a figure of 3% male practitioners has the highest percentage of such midwives in Europe.

Midwifery, the profession of being a "sage-femme", that is a confidante and comforter in the bloody business of existence and not just a woman who knows the pelvic mechanics, is one of the oldest professions, and certainly one of the very few dominated by women. And women are the largely the persons who educate society's infants, a word for children before they learn speech.

Men have long been both afraid of and grudgingly respectful of those who assist parturient women at this most dramatic moment. The first men who tried to commandeer this educational task were, as Ivan Illich remarked, bishops leading their flocks to the "alma ubera" (milk-brimming breasts) of the Mother Church, "from which they were never to be weaned." Jules Michelet in the mid-nineteenth century sought to take the side of the "mammana" in his book *La Sorcière*, but already the ancestral and even folkloric skills and practices of the midwife were being displaced in the United Kingdom and other European countries in favour of forceps-aided delivery techniques performed by a "man-midwife," otherwise known as an accoucheur or obstetrician. The best known in literature is Sterne's grotesque

Dr Slop, who is based on William Smellie, one of the celebrated man-midwives of the eighteenth century: he failed to appeal to all his female counterparts, one of them (Elizabeth Nihell) describing him memorably as a "great horse God-mother of a he-midwife."

In the 1990s, I used to read articles in French medical gazettes which advocated the adoption of the term *maïeuticien* to describe this seemingly new profession. There were objections to its use however, and they didn't come from sages-femmes. (Male) public intellectuals objected to such a dignified term being used to describe such a humble profession: maieutics in philosophy is a form of pedagogy that goes back to Socrates, whose ability to dissociate propositions from the circumstances of their origin made his resemble a midwife's art—dialectics being applied to determine whether the newly born idea was really a live birth. (Yet philosophy's beginnings were humble: in *Meno*, simply by asking questions, Socrates enables an uneducated slave boy to light upon a geometrical paradigm.)

Jacques Lacan, for one, had in his own lurid way long been promoting maieutics in an anti-Socratic sense: he wasn't so much exposing the presumption of those who think they know (but are actually ignorant) as offering help to those who suffer of the fact that they know, but don't know they know. (It is astonishing to think that the former American Secretary of State Donald Rumsfield had a direct line to the great French obfuscator.)

But didn't the historian Fernand Braudel portray modern France, with only a trace of sarcasm, as having received her final shape from the "cosmic midwifery" of the 1789 revolution?

CARELESS

"But I wish you to be without care." I remember this line from the Apostle Paul's most explicit instructions for living the messianic life, now that "time is straitened" (1 Cor. 7:29); and wonder if my own insouciance isn't a reaching back to my early understanding of these passages, which saturated my childhood. Being free of care was in fact the contrary of the charged atmosphere surrounding me, which was electric with worry and dread.

Giorgio Agamben notes that the Apostle Paul's famous passage about the straitening of time collapses the equally famous passage in Ecclesiastes (3:4-8) in which the Preacher makes a clear distinction between the times for weeping and laughing, mourning and dancing...

WELL-PERSON CLINICS

Many people, it would seem, think health is an appurtenance unto life, a blithe state of being which ought to be maintained and certified ISO9002. The car service metaphor is ubiquitous. But health has never carried this meaning. In fact, we readily confuse health with the ideology which has been rampant throughout the twentieth century: *fitness*.

Medicine as a humanism would seem doomed when people think of taking their bodies in—by analogy with the need to ensure that a car remains roadworthy—for service. The human body isn't a car however, and not only because it has self-healing and regenerating properties. Discerning consumer-patients aren't happy with a few words of reassurance from their personal doctor (an old-fangled notion), or a few practical tips on how to get "better"; they now want to be dealer-serviced by specialists.

PIG IGNORANCE

The decision to call the strain of influenza A (N1H1) doing the rounds in 2009 *swine* flu was not without consequences. Certainly the strain might have been first identified among pigs, but the illness is now a human influenza: it is spread person-to-person, and does not require intimate contact with infected animals, as does the N1H5 or "bird flu" strain, isolated human cases of which have been seen over the last five years in South East Asia.

The decision (in April 2009) by the Egyptian government— which incidentally imports fully one half of its caloric consumption, mostly in the form of American wheat and soya—to cull the 400 000 pigs kept in the country as a precautionary measure was widely criticised: no pigs in the country had been infected, nor can influenza be caught from pork that is properly prepared. As the French historian Michel Pastoureau reminds us in his cultural history of the pig *Le Cochon: Histoire d'un cousin mal aimé*, humans have always been exceptionally beastly towards the animal with which we genetically have most in common. Even before the genetic era, doctors knew that *Sus scrofa domesticus* was pretty much like us internally: one of Galen's most famous experiments involved cutting through a pig's recurrent laryngeal nerve: this particular pig continued to struggle to free itself from the wooden frame in which it was pinned but had lost its ability to squeal.

Our attitude to the pig has always been ambivalent. Jews and Muslims are notably averse to pork and even Christianity had its Gadarene moment—with its uncanny echo of the mystic rooting pigs of the Eleusinian mysteries. Perhaps only the long-civilised Chinese recognise the true human value of pigs, having almost half as many on their soil as humans. Whether they treat them properly or even allow them a reek of that soil is another matter. As Brett Mizelle observes, "the more pigs there are in the world, the harder it has become to see them". In fact, to see pigs raised outdoors you have to go to New Guinea or the South Sea islands, where on a Sunday morning many years ago I saw several plumes of smoke arising from the subterranean ovens in which the creatures that only the day before had been foraging around the guesthouse were being slowly baked.

In Europe the pig's interest in sniffing the soil made it unpopular with medieval clerics, who thought it evidence of devilishness; yet small children have an almost instinctive affection for pigs: indeed, nothing resembles the newborn child as much as a piglet. The elevation of the dog to the status of domestic animal, according to Pastoureau, meant that some of its instinctive rutting behaviour patterns had to be projected onto another animal: hence the French expression "faire des cochonneries"—to be dirty or smutty, especially in the sexual sense. Walter Burkert suggests that, in ancient Greece, pigs were linguistically associated with the female genitalia. The great blusterer Thomas Carlyle gave the name "pig-philosophy" to the reductive belief of his time under which humans were regarded as mere appetite-gratifying creatures rather than creatures endowed with a soul. Perhaps the projection was as much to deflect attention away from what humans themselves really like to get up to—or down to. It has even been rumoured that the ancient Semites had reasons other than hygienic for proscribing pork: its taste, according to the few experts on the subject, is remarkably similar to that of human flesh. One of the queasiest moments in William Golding's *Lord of the Flies* comes after the striplings have killed a pig and stuck its head on a pole. The pig's head, abuzz with flies, seems to speak to Simon: "You knew, didn't you? I'm part of you? Close, close, close! I'm the reason why it's no go? Why things are what they are?"

But in the bestiary of unpopular animals—which would include wolves, toads, crows, cats at one time, and of course goats—it is always the pig which is the first culprit. Egypt has a population of 80 million people crammed into a very small area of cultivable land: the Nile Valley and its delta account for only about four percent of its surface area. But that is not its only problem. Most of the pig handlers in the country are Copts. So too are the rubbish collectors of the ancient city of Cairo, *zabbaleen*, who are packed into a vast slum in the Moqattan Hills Settlement east of Cairo. For eighty years the zabbaleen have been collecting rubbish from at least one-third of Cairo's 14 million people free of charge, sorting it, and selling the organic waste to the pig farms.

Six months after the slaughter of the pigs the streets of Cairo were piled high with rubbish. The zabbaleen had become poorer than ever. They had been robbed of their livelihood. The pigs were in fact a major part of the extended relationships in Cairo's informal public garbage disposal system: the zabbaleen cleared the streets of rubbish, and sold their ordure to the pig farmers, whose pigs recycled it. Not only did the municipalities benefit from their services, the whole process was a very sophisticated and efficient one: most Western garbage collecting companies only recycle about 25 percent of their waste; in Cairo that figure was 80 percent. Some of the zabbaleen even invested in methods for recycling metal, glass, paper and fabrics. Now the pig farmers have gone bankrupt, the zabbaleen have nobody to sell their rubbish to. "They killed the pigs," said a former garbage collector, "let them clean the city."

Ancient professionalism

Hippocrates (460-377 BC), whose name means "horse-tamer", was the founder of a medical school on the island of Kos, and although it is doubtful whether he is the author of all sixty treatises that bear his name he has become known as the founder of the Hippocratic corpus. The promissory part of that tradition, the famous Hippocratic Oath, assumed that aspiring doctors would serve for several years as apprentices, usually while lodging with their masters. Thereupon would follow a period of peregrination, when young doctors would journey from city to city, sharpening and selling their skills, before settling down.

The corpus contains a treatise on environmental medicine called *Airs, Waters and Places* which was designed as a guide to help the novice practitioner establish a flourishing practice: on arriving in a new city, he is instructed to spend time getting used to the new surroundings, learning about the water supply and prevailing winds, and also about the lifestyle of the inhabitants. Another treatise stipulates that the physician's best selling point is himself, and tells doctors to make sure they were plump "as nature intended [them] to be"—clean, well-dressed and nice-smelling. A serious but not solemn demeanour is essential.

The doctor's booth in the marketplace ("surgery") ought to be sheltered but bright enough to allow proper treatment. Bronze furnishings are vulgar, but this metal happens to be the best for medical instruments. Instructions are given for deflecting criticism and especially for avoiding negligence: being convinced that one has a mission or even a pressing need to heal others is treated as a potential source of hubris, or at least a pretension sometimes deserving of ridicule.

Freud's debt to Nietzsche

The bitter ironies and self-excoriation of Nietzsche's style and way of thinking are a tacit recognition of the all-consuming nature of his thought, which undermined the belief that persons are knowable and consistent. It was in fact Sigmund Freud, a plump randy Watson to Nietzsche's thinly dangerous Holmes, who got the credit for developing a guild-controlled method for dealing out drops of the corrosive tincture that ate away at Nietzsche's innards.

"Trust me, I'm a doctor!" The price of his poison is that every psychoanalytic patient turns into a Hamlet. And if these stand-in Hamlets cared to read Nietzsche, they would discover that the Freudian notion of a "core self" mostly formed early in life and able to be "therapied" back into a reasonably functioning life, if not "liberated" entirely, is completely undermined by Nietzsche, who denies the reality of the self as an agent or subject in its own right ("'the doer' is merely a fiction added to the deed—the deed is everything" (*zur Genealogie der Moral*)).

Pity this

Originally "pitiful" was an adjective describing the person who expressed pity—one was full of pity just as one might be full of piety (and often the two went hand in hand). The Bible too talks of a pitiful God. In the sixteenth century the adjective underwent a complete reversal of sense and became associated with the object or person arousing or deserving of pity, that is to say *pitiable*, before becoming a modern term of deprecation, being almost synonymous with *abject, pathetic* or even *contemptible*.

The deeper sense of this shift in freight illustrates the fact that pity is a vertical, top-down emotion: the object of pity is deficient in some respect, and the person feeling pity condescends in the very acknowledgement of that lack. There can be no pity without a measure of contempt.

Which is why so many moral philosophers have written—

in opposition to Jean-Jacques Rousseau, who made it the primordial virtue—that we ought to prefer compassion to pity, since compassion (as its etymology suggests) asks you to venture a sidelong glance at your suffering neighbour. Compassion is the great Asiatic virtue of horizontal feeling.

THE SECRET

The more open doctors are about what they do, about being reps for a secular Eden and on occasion even pushers of a kind of desacralised Eucharist, and the more insistent they are about emancipating their patients from their self-imposed minority, the more resentment about this state of affairs is heightened, and the more the institution of medicine itself gets blamed for it.

Patients have come to believe that they are heartfelt and sincere and look askance when their doctor turns out to be a sceptic and a stickler for the facts.

DON'T TORTURE THAT INSTRUMENT!

Many people know the phrase Novalis committed to his notebook, "Every illness is a musical problem—the cure is a musical solution. The more rapid, and yet more complete the solution—the greater the musical talent of the doctor."

Novalis is reminding us of the ancient dispute about the principles of action at a distance and action by direct contact which survives in modern electromagnetic and quantum theory. Pythagoras knew that a string plucked close to another tuned to the same pitch would cause the second to vibrate in sympathy. The mathematical basis of harmony was based on the subdivisions of that string. Resonance therefore became a potent symbol of the relations of sympathy which bound the world together; it is the working principle of that beautiful baroque instrument, the viola d'amore, which, even in its name, was used to celebrate the mysterious attraction which had lovers trembling with mutual desire.

In his set of three philosophical dialogues, *Le Rêve d'Alambert*, Diderot considered the plucked strings of the harpsichord as an analogy for his understanding of the animal-machine (and his Jesuit friend Louis Bertrand Castel even devised an "ocular clavecin", for which Telemann wrote some pieces). David Hume also took up the harmonic potential of the nervous system in his *Treatise of Human Nature* (1740), when he adopted the new perceptual system proposed and systematised by Newton and Locke. The affections generated among human creatures, Hume thought, were like the sounds transmitted by musical instruments: we are "taken out of ourselves" because our pains and pleasures vibrate like so many violins with those of others. Their strings could be wound up and out of tune, or even overstretched and jittery. Adam Smith's philosophy of sympathy for the new mercantile world that was springing up around them is clearly indebted to this musico-tensile understanding of physiology. Even Edmund Burke thought rest helped to restore the tone of the "fibres" and half a century later Thomas Beddoes the physician imagined after sniffing nitrous oxide that he was composed of "finely vibrating strings." In modernist Vienna of the early twentieth century, the theorist Hermann Bahr went so far as to define the content of the new idealism as "nerves, nerves—and costume." When people today talk about being "a bundle of nerves", they're not thinking of those ordered fascicles of nerve fibres that course the body; they mean they're on edge and nervous, strings about to break.

Although the "strings" were metaphors called up by the new neurological understanding of man, the heart had acquired the most sensitive strings of all. Spencer had first used the term in a poem of 1596, when the tendons of heart muscle were mistaken for a kind of pulley system. "Admirable mechanism!" wrote Ann Radcliffe. "All the other strings of the heart vibrate when that of humanity has just been sounded." And it was precisely as sentimental literature was developing as a leisure form that cultivated people were beginning to enjoy performances on the harpsichord and violin, and not long before the piano would be introduced to households considerably further down the social scale.

Yet behind this angelic statement about the healing skills of music stands the bloody story of the defeat of Marsyas, the pipe player, by Apollo, the god whose lyre was the purer instrument. He was harmony's surgeon.

Funeral practices

Sarcasm, from the Greek *sarkazein*: to separate the flesh from the bones. Or perhaps more pointedly, to mock a corpse (*sarx*), which is unable to object to our act of contumely.

Against decomposition

Epidemics exist in three dimensions at the same time: in the larger environment outside the human body, in actual organised physical bodies, and in the varying set of relations we call the social body.

The essential thing to remember is that the first of these three is primordial, in both senses of the word. Animals are the intruders in a world of micro-organisms: primitive bacteria were present on Earth 3.5 billion years ago, in the aeon known as the Proterozoic, long before more complex lifeforms emerged; that our cells are themselves composite structures incorporating archaic bacteria that have become commensal (mitochondria); and that within minutes of birth a baby's mucosa is carpeted with billions of microbes most of which will be beneficial to the future welfare of the child (the gut microbiome). Our social life is indebted to these silent precursors: respiration, photosynthesis and fermentation all rely on micro-organisms. Less than one percent of bacteria are pathogens.

Epidemics jolt us into recalling how much of what we call *life* is subterranean, mysterious and invisible: the "return of the repressed" is actually the often terrified realisation that how we think our bodies are organised has almost nothing to do with their true physiological and molecular nature. Death, from the microbial perspective, is to enter a different metabolic and compositional state.

Epidemics prompt us to recompose the details and manner of our social life, and remind us that the vulnerability of apparently solid bodies is also an inherent aspect of vitality itself.

Being kind

A doctor whose opinions I greatly esteem, and whose religious upbringing was similar to my own, recently wrote in his personal newsletter about the benefits of medicalising anxiety and shyness (and other problems) "if it helps people", and finished his comment by suggesting that such a trend can be seen either "as a sinister triumph of disease-mongering, or just the way we have to deal with things in a society which for all its faults is steadily getting kinder."

Two things struck me about his assertion: that perhaps only someone who grew up in decent, tranquil, socialised, middle-class, post-war England could have expressed such an indolently benevolent view of the way we have to deal with things; and that bowdlerising is still a strong impulse, perhaps stronger now even than in the Victorian era. As the Bhagavad Gita insists, in the name of all those ancient Asian societies that neither strive nor even pretend to be kind, this world is ultimately one in which we eat and are eaten. Simone Weil says this too. But my colleague was right in the sense that the grounds for partiality and inequity, because they cannot be eradicated, now have to be *explained* to those who suffer them; and this new understanding of the public good then becomes enshrined in legal statutes. But perhaps "kinder" is not the right word.

Terminator ethics

Medicine cannot get away ethically from the face-to-face. That must be agony for some people, as they feel themselves by the minute become anachronisms of a more humane—or at least a more civil—age.

Telling the truth to power

The disturbing story of the German neurologist Edmund Forster, as related in Ernst Weiss' novel *The Eyewitness*: he is supposed to have treated Adolf Hitler in the last month of the Great War for the symptoms of hysterical blindness. In 1933, after the Nazi takeover, he travelled to Paris to hand over details of the case to his diplomat brother (from whom Weiss is thought to have cribbed his novel) and returned to his professorial duties at the University of Greifswald with heavy forebodings. After being denounced by a student and undergoing interrogation by the Gestapo, he was found dead of a single gunshot wound in his bathroom. Forster was buried as a suicide. The records about Hitler's imaginary illness have never been traced, though one historian believes they were deposited in the vault of a Basel bank. Another, even more illustrious neurologist-psychiatrist Vladimir Behkterev, one of the first scientists to put forward the role of the hippocampus in memory formation and retention and describe the mechanism of the reflex arc, as well as to study the power of suggestion in the hypnotic seance ("the direct conveyance of ideas, emotions, or any other psychophysical conditions to another person's mind in such a way as to bypass his critical faculties"), was poisoned in 1927, shortly after having told Stalin that he was suffering from paranoia.

The fate of both these physicians contrasts markedly with that of Hitler's *Leibarzt* or personal physician, Theodor Morell, who was soundly disliked by everyone else in the dictator's entourage, most of whom thought him a quack; he kept "the great man" dosed to the eyeballs on a regimen of morphine, barbiturates, amphetamines and strychnine (to combat his flatulence), most of them delivered by injection. Morell enjoyed special favours as a type of Doctor Feelgood; but for both Forster and Behkterev frank diagnosis was an act of lèse-majesté, and the first citizen of both state cults spared nobody until he was sure that he had maintained the inviolability of his person.

A MORBID SENSITIVITY

It's a dubious benefit to have a thin skin. "Une sensibilité à fleur de peau", as the rather beautiful French expression has it, which conjures up one of those anatomical flayed men, so exposed to our regard he doesn't have a skin at all.

Many such hypersensitive people write books, which objects started their distinguished career in civilised life as the part product of flayed, stretched and treated animal skins. And people who write books tend to believe in Leonardo's prophecy "Of the Skins of Animals": "The more you converse with skins covered over with sentiments, the more you will acquire wisdom".

That's why Bartholomew the Apostle (sentenced to death by flaying) is the patron saint of tanners, tailors, leatherworkers, butchers and bookbinders. Artisans who can stomach the sour smell of leather and mordant.

Always at a loss

Oliver Sacks' book *Musicophilia* made me think of Jorge Luis Borges' famous story "Funes the Memorious". Borges tells of a teenage Uruguayan boy who suffers a horseback riding accident and ends up a cripple. The accident has had a strange outcome: Funes is immobilised but "now his perception and memory [are] infallible." He tells the narrator about his feats of memory, perceiving the shapes of clouds at any given moment, reconstructing a whole day (which would take him a day) and devising absurd infinite vocabularies for natural numbers: he can forget nothing. He is consequently incapable of generalities or abstractions, is constantly surprised by his own face in the mirror, or the movements of beings in space: "he was the solitary and lucid spectator of a multiform, instantaneous and almost intolerably precise world."

Sacks's book is also full of people who have suffered similar accidents and emerged with curious, in this case, musical abilities. One orthopaedic surgeon is struck by lightning on the way home. He seems to recover but then a few weeks later has an intense, all-consuming desire to listen to piano music, something he had never experienced before. Soon he is teaching himself to play, hearing music in his head, noting down the melodies that come to him unbidden, driving his wife crazy with impromptu concerts. As Sacks says, musicality seems to be a human ability that can accompany low intelligence and poor linguistic abilities, and blindness appears to favour a compensatory growth of the auditory sphere. But it's never clear in his book what counts as music. Is it rhythm, or melody, or something structural... and why aren't musical scales universal? Nevertheless, it's a surprise to learn that Nabokov was tone-deaf: he once wrote that music affected him "merely as an arbitrary succession of more of less irritating sounds." Sacks himself seems deaf to types of music other than classical: he certainly doesn't groove.

There is no obvious evolutionary reason why most of us would agree with Nietzsche that life without music is a mistake. Courtship display looks a bit odd if you take Wagner's *Liebestod* as your example. Some of the people in Sacks' book suffer from extreme amnesia yet still retain songs from their childhood. Musical memory goes deep into the sense of self, and it can modulate involuntary tics and chorea into coherence. Anyone who has nursed a demented relative will know the power of music to act on the personality that has taken leave of its surroundings. In fact, what comes across most obviously, in a book like this, is that neurology is a privative discipline—or, as Sacks has written elsewhere, "deficit is its favourite word". While it knows how to define loss and deficit it finds it much more difficult to define and conceptualise its opposite, surfeit or excess. Our brains are far more plastic than we have thought, and perhaps need to be reined in; until, as is the case with Funes, we hit our head on a rock and start to think we can keep the entire world in mind.

Folie à deux

It is part of contemporary allopathic medicine's self-image that it is perfectly upstanding and righteous and completely remote from the kind of snake-oil marketing that used to hang around its nearly worthless proprietary products in the Victorian age. The public accept the image at face value too. Everybody basks in the glow. But it is striking that what were formerly rare and debilitating diseases have now become lifestyle options. Since we have designer individualism designer drugs should hardly surprise us: diseases have in fact been restyled to sell medications. And everybody stands to benefit. One of the central aspects of the whole conundrum is that doctors tend to attribute beneficial changes in a patient's condition to their own actions, while overlooking any possible harm. Enthusiasm (i.e. being inspired or possessed by a god) is what really makes patients better. This bias is so ingrained they fail to notice it. And the mere fact that doctors *say* they mean to do good largely exonerates them when things go wrong. And the pharmaceutical industry has taken infinite pains to ask doctors what matters most to them, and then marketed those things back to them. In economic terms, it is doctors who act as primary recipients of the consumer message, although they do not take the drugs they prescribe. They believe they have an explicative advantage over their patients but they themselves are maximally explicated by the industry, with its huge marketing departments.

The whole sorry thing could almost be described as a *struggle of competing naiveties*.

CUTTING OFF YOUR NOSE

You can't *olfactorise* in a manner that would offer any meaningful parallel with the active sense according to the verb *visualise*, but you can certainly *odorise*. Or even better *de-odorize*, which seems to be one of the chief contributions of North American society to the history of civilised behaviour.

PRESUMPTIONS

Some of my doctor colleagues used to claim to be able to diagnose what was wrong with their patients as soon as they entered the consulting room—like the head waiter in the finest restaurant in Prague in Borumil Hrabal's novel *I Served the King of England*, who astounds his protégé by anticipating exactly what guests will order immediately on their sitting down at table. "Isn't it horrifying to think that a careful observer can discover a vice, a twinge of remorse, a disease, just by looking at a man walking," wrote Balzac in 1830. The Edinburgh physician Dr Joseph Bell, on whom Arthur Conan Doyle based his character Sherlock Holmes, would "sit in his receiving room... and diagnose the people as they came in, before they even opened their mouths. He would tell them details of their past lives; and hardly would he ever make a mistake."

Certainly, some physical postures may well give valuable clues towards diagnosis, such as altered gait or demeanour, and there is the acetone smell of diabetes and the pathognomonic appearance of certain diseases (e.g. the rash associated with Lyme disease), but it usually takes a few words before doctors can start to apply the heuristics of clinical reasoning. The tradition of being ahead of yourself seems to have a long pedigree: Galen, the great Roman physician of Greek origin, was already claiming that he could "read" patients—sometimes "at a glance." Oliver Sacks in his autobiography *On the Move* tells of his boss at the Middlesex Hospital, Michael Kremer, who was "intuitive in the extreme", and could diagnose rare disorders as soon as a newly admitted patient entered the ward: Kremer wrote a paper called "Sitting, Standing, and Walking" which detailed how much could be understood before a routine neurological exam or indeed before the patient had said a word.

Patients are—unsurprisingly—none too keen on being "read at a glance" by a prim physician, although the likelihood of such an inferred reading is high, even when the doctor lacks the diagnostic skills of a Galen or Kremer: some studies show that the average doctor interrupts a patient's opening gambit after 18-23 seconds. The impulse to diagnose and categorise clearly runs up hard against the notion that listening might be a therapeutic act in its own right.

In this respect, the generally sympathetic bond of general practice flouts the grounding principles of psychoanalysis, where the person-to-person encounter is the important part of the therapeutic relationship: the analyst's expertise is above all a particularly attentive kind of listening, although the analytical encounter is sometimes just as far from being a conversation as the abrupted medical presentation. Some psychoanalysts have been known to sit though an analysis without uttering a single word, a supposedly transference-preventing strategy which would surely unnerve most (if not all) patients.

It would seem then that the person "presenting" in both types of encounter is peculiarly exposed.

In the hypothetico-deductive model, one or two causal notions are generated early in the consultation and the evidence then sifted against the familiar patterns of disease presentation. This kind of reasoning is both intuitive and analytical, and has been shown to be the best way to arrive at a working diagnosis, though of course the practical need to terminate proceedings within a reasonable time and the bias of considering only those data that reinforce the original hypothesis can skew its predictive power. Medical students cautiously heap up data obtained through investigations long before formulating a diagnosis. Many mature doctors on the other hand have learned, partly through its effects on themselves, that time is the most valuable diagnostic tool. (And it shouldn't be forgotten that about one-third of all presentations of illness in practice entail what have been called "medically unexplained symptoms.")

To comfort my colleagues I used to tell them that Luis Buñuel, the provocative Spanish film director, liked to imagine a little algorithmic device that would be able to predict the ending of every Hollywood movie based on information provided by the first few scenes. All the same, I couldn't help but recall Dostoyevski's Father Zossima in *The Brothers Karamazov* who "could see directly into the souls of other people": Wittgenstein told his pupil Rush Rhees that because Zossima had listened to so many people baring their hearts and asking for advice "in the end he had acquired so fine a perception that he could tell at a glance from the face of a stranger what he had come for, what he wanted and what kind of torment racked his soul."

It is a disconcerting thought, however, that if the "souls of other people" are removed from the setting, person-reading seems remarkably akin to behaviourism, first made popular by the American psychologist John B. Watson in 1928: he simply denied that consciousness existed—life could be explained as the doings of so many automatons. "Our accomplishments, even our words and sentences, are so limited and stereotyped that you can pretty well predict what the majority of men and women are going to say and do in most situations. We are so stupidly uninteresting." So wrote the founder of a paradoxical psychology without a psyche, although Watson had to exempt himself from his own argument in order to validate its thesis.

The converse of this instant diagnosis model is the reminiscence in his memoirs by Elias Canetti of his Russian friend, the remarkable short story writer Isaac Babel, who returned from exile in France to the Soviet Union. Babel was eventually killed in 1940 by the NKVD after a difficult decade in which he was first criticised for low productivity and then sidelined: at the first congress of the Union of Soviet Writers (1934), he had noted ironically that he was becoming "the master of a new literary genre, the genre of silence." Babel, writes Canetti, "taught me a way of looking at people: gazing at them for a long time, as long as they were to be seen, without breathing a single word about what you saw… I learned from him that one can gaze for a very long time without knowing, that one can tell only much later whether one knows something about a person: after losing sight of him."

In other words, as Gabriel Josipovici says, in his great study of the Bible as a book: "We do not decipher people, we encounter them."

COLOURS OF THE WORKING WEEK

The blue of the sky was the topic of the conversation Elliott Felkin had with Thomas Hardy in 1919, and which he recounted in a 1962 issue of *Encounter* magazine. "He went on to talk about days of the week and colours and associations. Monday was colourless, and Tuesday a little less colourless, and Wednesday was blue—'this sort of blue' pointing to an imitation Sèvres plate—and Thursday is a darker blue, and Friday is dark blue, and Saturday is yellow, and Sunday is always red…". We can take it that Hardy was not thrilled with his Mondays, nor even his Tuesdays; but that things really started humming with the prospect of something Chinese or cerulean midweek, and weekends were decidedly shrill compared to the resonant *basso profondo* of Friday.

Parallel worlds

Medicine is only a step away from a kind of metaphysics. Prevention involves acting to ensure that an unwanted possibility is relegated to the ontological realm of non-actualised possibilities. Yet the unwanted event, even though it is now unlikely to occur, retains its status as a special kind of hypothetical event, not so much in the sense that it is still a possibility (for that is what we have acted to hinder) but that in some unexplorable future anterior *it could still have happened*.

And perhaps medicine is then only a step away from a kind of madness.

Finger to mouth

Here is a party question. If you had to lose a finger, which one do you think you could do best without? Most people will guess the small finger, which is wrong. Bioengineers and evolutionists tell us that in the extraordinarily complex functional anatomy of the hand, in which the hypermobile human thumb interacts with the other fingers and allows humans unparalleled dexterity and power, it is the index finger that is least important, not least since we can still hold a pen and fork without it.

I'm not so sure. These engineers of the human frame are overlooking (as evolutionists tend to do) the importance of the index finger in ostensive language, or definition-by-pointing: it is the pointing finger which advertises by analogy the importance of language in human development. You understand the rule without even thinking about it—otherwise, as Wittgenstein noted in *Philosophical Investigations*, you would look all the way up the pointing person's arm.

Ethical poles

Philip Larkin thought it obvious that "self's the man." Emmanuel Levinas, a citizen of the nation that is structured socially on the basis of philosophical egoism, reduced his ethics to two words: "After you." Politeness towards others is a good basis for developing a moral sense, as every parent used to know, even though politeness is a virtue of pure form. For many people in our expressive and impulsive age a polite person is simply not an *authentic* person. Unashamedly looking after Number One seems to be a more honest undertaking. Contemporary educationalists remark on how self-esteem has been enthroned as the highest attribute of personhood, and anyone working in a public service knows that the idea of putting others first is often treated with derision and naked impatience.

Rabbi Hillel, two millennia ago in the Babylonian Talmud, had already pondered this dilemma: "If I'm not for myself, who will be? But if I'm only for myself, who am I?" In some cultures, isolation is a living death: to be a person is understood as being part of a social configuration. In the words of the ancient Egyptian proverb: "One lives as one is led by another."

Depression and rational design

Tricyclic antidepressants emerged in the 1950s, at which time it was thought that no more than 50 to 100 people per million suffered the kind of depression that would respond to these new drugs; and the pharmaceutical companies saw no great interest in their development and marketing. Sales in the next decade were poor in comparison to the major and minor tranquillisers like the benzodiazepines—mockingly popularised as "mother's little helper" by the Rolling Stones in one of their songs. It was only with the arrival on the market of "rationally-designed" selective serotonin reuptake inhibitors in the 1980s, that antidepressants became big business: the use of antidepressants in the United States doubled in the decade between 1996 to 2005, by which year they were being prescribed to 27 million citizens; a similar rise was observed in the United Kingdom in the decade up to 2002 when their use increased by 234 percent. Significant percentages of people in the non-institutionalised population, i.e. ordinary persons, are taking an antidepressant drug. In 2020, the total world revenue for branded antidepressants is forecast to be over 16 billion dollars, although several famous proprietary products will have lost patent protection and become generics.

Despite all the evidence trotted out to convince doctors that they are diagnosing and treating a real bipolar disorder with or without mania or psychosis, and the methods of persuasion (sometimes government-sanctioned) deployed to convince patients to visit doctors in the first place, we need to remind ourselves that psychiatry is an intellectual construct. Its models are calqued on those of physical illness, and its explanations owe as much to verbal ingenuity as to hard facts or findings. How can anybody regard those figures and not suspect a monstrous complot, especially when we know now that the measurable effect of many of these SSRIs is barely distinguishable from that of a placebo?

That they might have life, and have it more abundantly

If health *is* a religion, then our life expectancy has been drastically diminished. We have only mere life to look forward to, while our ancestors had the prospect of more life as the consummation of their earthly sojourn. And the spectacular mass vitalism of consumption has managed to hide from us the fact that our striving for things we already have is a withering and sad symptom of a deeper need. As Karl Kraus wrote, "you don't even live once." (Which is truly witty in the original German: "Sie leben nicht einmal einmal".)

Take Rabelais' advice

Fly from those men, that great rabble of false-cenobites, hooded cheats, sluggards, hypocrites, canters, tub-thumpers, monks in boots, and other sects of people; never trust in men who peer from under a cowl.

An ectoparasite from the Cretaceous

I became familiar with a new disease vector when I was in practice in Strasbourg: the ixodids.

Every spring in the woods of Europe thousands of people (and other vertebrates) get bitten by ticks (*Ixodes ricinus*). I once watched, horrified, after a daylong walk in the Vosges as an entire family of juvenile ticks, tinier even than poppy seeds, quested their way up my trouser leg; and have over the years had to remove swollen sessile ticks from the limbs of patients, family members, and various parts of my own anatomy. Gentle but steady traction is needed to remove the ticks intact along with their hypostome or holdfast organ, an ingenious reverse-toothed harpoon-like structure that anchors them while feeding. Most tick bites, which generally go undetected (due to chemicals called "evasins"), cause no more than a little local redness; a few can be the source of a number of diseases, the best known of which is Lyme disease or borreliosis, an infection caused by a spirochete (*Borrelia burgdorferi*). It is generally easily treatable with antibiotics, provided patients present the pathognomonic or telltale sign of erythema chronicum migrans (a circular rash expanding from the bite site until it resembles a "bull's eye"). As with so many diseases however, there are always variants and sometimes "silent" exceptions. If it goes undiagnosed, borreliosis can cause cardiological, rheumatological and neurological problems at a much later date.

Ticks also transmit viral infections: I used to vaccinate patients who liked to go hill-walking in eastern Europe, where tick-borne encephalitis is relatively common: it is also transmitted more rapidly, whereas the borrelia spirochetes are activated by the blood meal and need time to accumulate in the tick mouthparts. The further east you go, towards the Balkans and the Crimea, the more severe these viral infections can be: some are haemorrhagic and carry high mortality rates.

The more I learned about ticks the more fascinated I became. To say that they are understudied is an understatement: it was only in the late 1970s, when I went to medical school, that Lyme disease was formally described. Tests are rarely requested, and often not available, for some of the other diseases transmitted by ticks, such as babesiosis (caused by a protozoon that infects red blood cells) or anaplasmosis (a rickettsial illness).

When you consider their life cycle it is hardly surprising ticks are implicated in zoonoses—diseases transmitted between animals and humans. An adult female tick can lay up to 3000 eggs: the eggs then go through successive developmental stages from larva to nymph to imago (adult). Ticks are obligate parasites: each of the three development stages requires at least one blood meal over several days. Since each meal will be taken from a different host the potential for ticks to acquire hitchhiking microbes is very high. The entire developmental cycle usually lasts about three years, although it can be longer depending on climatic conditions. Ticks are found on every continent, but prefer warm moist conditions, precisely the kind of conditions ecologists say are likely to become more common in the northern hemisphere with global warming.

The French philosopher Gilles Deleuze, in his series of speculations on "le devenir-animal", tried to grasp the limited experience of the tick's world, which is clearly the reason for its success as a parasite. Its three "excitations" are to crawl to the tip of a branch or twig, to sense an immediate animal presence (which it does by means of Haller's organ, a structure on its front legs that reacts to environmental and olfactory stimuli), and once established on its host to perforate the skin. What is extraordinary about the tick is that it can bide its time, obdurately, for months or even years, to ambush a warm-blooded animal. Another philosopher, Giorgio Agamben, instanced a tick that had survived for 18 years in a Rostock laboratory without being nourished or even stimulated as one of his models of "bare life".

It would be surprising if this ancient arachnid—seemingly no more than a mouthpiece with attached legs and body—were not to be associated with emerging diseases in the twenty-first century.

Signe d'appel

The French surgeon René Leriche is famous for his phrase "the silence of the body," meaning that the body generally gives few clues as to the illnesses it is incubating.

Most people, I think, would be surprised to hear that a physician would ever think the body *silent*—in the primary sense of being noiseless and uncommunicative.

What Leriche was recouping was the observation made long before him by the philosopher Immanuel Kant that while we can *feel* ourselves to be in perfect health, we can never *know* that we are.

Total liability

I have seen it attested that in ancient Egypt and in some of the Mesopotamian societies, the attending physician was subject to total liability—which meant that if the patient died, the doctor lost his life too. This seems most implausible, for obvious reasons. Nevertheless, it does suggest a certain kind of anthropological levelling—the doctor ought to suffer if he is unable to relieve the suffering he claimed to be able to treat in the first place: he couldn't have been much of a doctor, so deserves to die for being an impostor.

Whose will was paramount in the whole business? The punishment would make it seem the doctor had forced himself on his patient. But could a mere doctor be a god? Should he aspire to such a status? Clearly, if he did, then there might be something permissible about stoning him to death for failing to exert the aforementioned godlike powers.

Medical humanity

It is a peculiar (if understandable) *déformation professionnelle* of doctors to imagine their role in their patients' lives to be greater than it is. Doctors don't confer or deliver health to their patients. Health is an attribute of the individual person, not something that is handed over—like a bottle of pills—by a doctor. If a patient comes in with a health problem, doctors ought to be asking how they can help the patient surmount the problem and get on with life, not dwell on the matter as it were something of terrible moment.

The advantage of a cold eye

Here is Jane Austen's dry and abrasively honest comment in a letter (31 May, 1811) after reading about a battlefield scene in the Peninsular War: "How horrible it is to have so many people killed! And what a blessing that one cares for none of them!"

Today such frankness would be considered evidence of total heartlessness. She would be called a cold fish (and worse). But we know Jane Austen wasn't heartless; she was a novelist, after all. She was equally a rigorous thinker and knew where she stood in relation to events. Emotions were not to be cheaply indulged. We might say Jane Austen had a clear sense of "values", except that she would not have put the word in this context. "Values" only came into common use in the twentieth century when we became reluctant to use moral terms, not least because the approbation and censure that often accompanies them was regarded as a sign of intolerance—and nothing is a more obvious contemporary moral failing than intolerance.

What Jane Austen would have used was the word "virtue", now almost an archaism except among moral philosophers. Alasdair MacIntyre, for one, has described her novels as "the last great representative of the classical tradition of virtues." And indeed, if you look closer at the words, there is a gulf between virtues and values: virtues reside in what a person does, values—

so often economic in nature—are generated by the act of valuing. The noun is a function of the verb. We now use the term "value-neutral" but values themselves are neutral in the sense that they allow us to comment on another person's actions without feeling bound by our evaluations. Values are slippery and relativistic. Edward Skidelsky makes the distinction clear by referring to an extreme case: "We can speak of Nazi values without ourselves being taken for Nazis—something we cannot do if we speak of Nazi virtues."

The term "caring"—as Skidelsky observes in a related article in his column "Words that think for us" in *Prospect* magazine—is a term that only became common in the last half of the twentieth century. Dying soldiers anywhere merit compassion and concern, and the imagination recoils at scenes of slaughter, but there is no meaningful way we can care for unknown others. Care in the nineteenth century implied a relationship of guardianship, and very specific, often physically onerous responsibilities; it wasn't that contemporary flag for benevolence—a caring person now being just about as virtuous as it is possible to be (suggesting that while the virtues are deeply unfashionable we are more concerned than ever about looking good and ranking others). In fact, Austen is very clear about it being a *blessing* that we care for none of them. In fact, she uses the impersonal pronoun "one" (which—significantly—has become almost archaic too) to make the absence of the moral obligation even clearer. The awareness that she bears no physical proximity or relationship to the killed allows her to go on living. She doesn't make a scene because the scene is elsewhere.

Her comment is commonsensical and English, and a long time before anyone ever had the notion that displaying concern and distress in public could be interpreted as signs of virtuousness. "We frequently feel less than we are supposed to feel," wrote Craig Raine in an article about the artist Ron Mueck. "Or feel it differently. Or adulterated with 'inappropriate' feelings."

"Inappropriate", as Skidelsky notices, is another of those weasel words that signals how we ought to think and feel about others.

A word to stand by

The multiple origins of words in the English language have left some curious linguistic relics: homonyms or near-homonyms of different origin ("repair", "pawn", etc.). The first definition of the verb *cure* supplied by the OED is "to take care of; to care for: intr. to take trouble, to take care – 1623" which it derives from the Old French *curer*, related to the Latin *curare*. The substantive was taken up into the Catholic and Anglican office of "the cure of souls"— the ministering to the everyday needs of the congregation. (The Latin base term, in the same century, also supplied the adjective "accurate", meaning to "act with care", not as painstaking as "exact" but stronger than merely "correct".)

The verb *care*, on the other hand, already embedded in the definition of cure (as above), actually has an entirely different developmental route. It came about from the Old English *carian*, "to sorrow or lament", "to feel concern or interest", and is an extension of the proto-Germanic *karo, which still haunts the contemporary German term for the Holy Week—"Karwoche"— when the life of Jesus became dramatically darker, although it has accreted a different sense in contemporary German through the adjective "karg" (meaning "meagre" or "sparing"). Care is a word with worry on its mind—a grief word, a stricken word.

In short, cure and care are only apparent cognates. Care in itself is no guarantee of a cure, but cure surely entails care. Care's true nature is revealed by another etymology: "to stand beside" is the original sense of the act of assistance, which is the very least we hope medical staff will provide (from the Latin "ad sistere").

A hard thing

Death has become such a hidden event that it is only too easy to consider it the natural preserve of doctors, nurses and professional disposers of bodies. Things were not always so. At the beginning of *The Notebooks of Malte Laurids Brigge*, Rilke imagines death in turn as a kind of hand-me-down ("They are happy if they find one that more or less fits...") or a Johnny Appleseed legend ("The children had a small one in them and the grownups a large one. The women had it in their womb and the men in their chest.").

Rilke was greatly attached to this idea of death not so much as a fatal outcome attached to a sickness, but as the meaning that settles around a life once it has stopped talking. He himself, before he died of leukaemia in 1926, remembered jabbing his thumb on a rose bush, and told his friends that the rose had done him to death. Hence his elegantly flowery epitaph, "rose, o pure rose of contradiction, no one's sleep under so many lids", which puns on his own given name "Reiner". His personal myth had been sealed.

His admired French coeval Paul Valéry was rather more dismissive about death, although he wrote about it now and again in his famous *Cahiers*. "Death is a living person's idea. It is terrifying because of the amount of life the living person invests in it." "Death speaks to us in a deep resonant voice—and says nothing." He was entirely unpersuaded by the old idea, which Montaigne made much of in his *Essays*, of philosophy as being above all a preparation for death (the last and most crucial essay, as it were). Valéry: "Of all thoughts, the most futile is that of death."

The American art critic and essayist Dave Hickey takes a grammatical view of the issue: "Death is sad, but it is not a bad thing. It's punctuation. It makes room for the kids."

The other consciousness

As François Roustang has pointed out, it is unfortunate that the phenomenon known as hypnosis was assimilated (by James Baird) to a Greek word that suggests it is a form of sleep. In fact, entering a trance is almost the opposite: it is a state of *hypervigilance*, the primary purpose of which is not to send the subject "over" (in spite of the sense of rest and relaxation that many subjects report after the trance has been lifted) but to "reinstall" the person in his or her body: the senses then deliver a stream of concentrated perceptive qualia that become available to imaginative consideration. Freud talked of a "widening of consciousness" but it more closely resembles a narrowing or focussing—or the heightening Gaston Bachelard called a "reverie" (which he distinguishes from a "daydream"). The role of language in this process is crucial: it serves as a mechanism for directing the selective attention of the subject.

In psychoanalysis, by contrast, the body is considered from an erotic or sexual angle—hence Freud's desire to rid psychoanalysis of hypnosis, and thereby "purify" what he considered the inevitable process of transference: he thought that although hypnosis often had a cathartic effect it was more important for patients not to avoid the harder task of gaining insight of the analytic kind into the sources of their mental conflicts.

Hochstapelei

The *British Medical Journal* reports on a 38-year-old "paranoid schizophrenic with psychosis" who managed to obtain a post as an Assistenzarzt in the Ubbo-Emmius Hospital in the city of Norden in Lower Saxony using forged documents which purported to show that he had qualified in medicine at the Donetsk National University in Ukraine. He was able to work from March 2016 until June 2017, employing the jargon and methods which had been used during his own treatment, at which point the medical registration body became suspicious about the authenticity of his documents. During his employment in Norden, charges were filed against him at a district court in Lower Saxony (and dropped because he was purportedly undergoing psychiatric treatment) regarding a previous episode in the period 2006-2011 when he claimed to be a trained elderly care nurse. He is now facing further charges of forgery and fraud in Hanover.

Impostors, as Thomas Mann knew, always bear some relationship to their historical era: they are the persons other people are looking for (but only they know it).

Poets and managers

It was that fecund poet, Guillaume Apollinaire, who wrote: "Already scientific language is in deep disagreement with the poets' language. It is an unbearable state for things to be in."

Then came the two cultures debate in 1959, with the publication of C.P. Snow's book in which he warned that "advanced Western society" was divided into two hostile groups at loggerheads with the other across "a gulf of mutual incomprehension". The debate must have struck a chord, since many people still remember Snow's role in this controversy (as if he had written nothing else), and the poet W.H. Auden was moved to reveal in his notes *The Poet & The City* that when he found himself in the company of scientists, he felt "like a shabby curate who has strayed by mistake into a drawing room full of dukes." Not all writers have had such an internalised sense of guilt about scientific language. As a leading lepidopterist, Nabokov was entitled to feel that he had all the qualifications and experience needed to move in both worlds (and then some): "I would have compared myself to a Colossus of Rhodes bestriding the gulf between the thermodynamics of Snow and the Laurentomania of Leavis, had that gulf not been a mere dimple of a ditch that a small frog could straddle."

In the early nineteenth century, the age of Goethe (who wrote on comparative anatomy, meteorology, geology, botany and morphology in addition to working over sixty years on *Faust*, his tremendous dramatic fable about a man obsessed with knowing and doing), there was no gulf between literature and science, since neither existed in the form we know them as today. It was a part of polite society to attend scientific experiments, with their marvels and mishaps. Literature, for Dr Johnson, was "learning; skill in letters," a broader field than today, and on the other side, there was no such thing as a "scientist". A *science* stood for any organised corpus of knowledge such as chemistry and theology, whereas medicine and engineering were *arts*. Sir Humphry Davy's lectures on chemistry at the Royal Institution in 1802 were a sensation at the time, and leading poets didn't think twice about attending them: Coleridge and Wordsworth were both in the auditorium.

It would seem as if the real debate now is not between science and poetry, for both make similar demands on the imagination, which is no respecter of social roles and the status quo, but between a culture open to imaginative endeavour in both spheres, and one in which all aspects of society are run on pseudo-scientific principles by people called *managers*, most of whose concepts stem from a once obscure offshoot of cybernetics called *systems theory*. The problem with the servomechanisms of systems theory is that users are always snarling up the loop. The mathematicians and social scientists attending the famous Macy Conferences in the 1940s and who devised systems theory were utterly convinced that it would foster peace across the globe and liberate humanity. Their assumption now seems a peculiarly unthinking compulsion—the shackled extension of a subjectless mythology of method. The key text here is Norbert Wiener's *The Human Use of Human Beings: Cybernetics and Society* (1950), the title of which is unabashed about its ambition.

An odd case

A general practitioner in this month's *British Journal of General Practice* wonders why so much money and attention is given to training doctors and nurses in basic life support techniques when it is uncommon for patients to succumb to cardiac arrests in GP surgeries. "It is probably pretty rare."

My first ever house visit as a GP trainee in Wigtownshire involved the successful resuscitation of a woman in her fifties who had been sitting at home with what she thought was abdominal pain all day. Just after I arrived with my trainer, she collapsed, pulseless, on her bed. She was in ventricular fibrillation. We ran back to the car boot, got out the defib, galvanised her heart back into sinus rhythm, telephoned the ambulance to take her to the local hospital; and she was back home in a week. Soon I had a reputation to live up to in the locality.

Of course, there was nothing statistically significant about the experience. But has anyone ever had a statistically significant experience?

Blighted hope

According to an article in the *Financial Times* there were no less than five stagings of *Uncle Vanya* in the United Kingdom this week (2013), confirming the remark made long ago by Kenneth Tynan that Chekhov's plays have been "remade in our image". What does that play speak of, if not of the steeping effects of time and the realisation of wasted potential? First Astrov, the local doctor, complains of the strains of his working life, and then Vanya, who, at 47, goes through a midlife crisis compounded by the arrival of his feckless brother-in-law, the pompous Professor Serebryakov and his beautiful younger wife Helen. Their arrival has upset the work routine. Outside it is raining, and inside everybody feels sorry for himself. "Soon the rain will be over. All living things will revive and breathe more freely. Except me."

Vanya has realised, twenty-five years too late, that he has been minding the estate of an academic fool, and that his own ambition and chances are spent. Underneath the non-events of the play there surges a feeling of panic, and the sense of time slipping through fingers. And that is drama enough.

How clever of Chekhov, who got to live only to the age of forty-four, to anticipate that the civilisation of the future would covet youth while ineluctably putting on girth.

"Thou art translated"

Some words don't mean what they say. Unbearable, for one. When you use it, the adjective doesn't allude to events that can't be put up with or endured. A literally unbearable event would have blasted you through the window of reality. What is "unbearable" is an existentially probing, even harrowing, situation.

As Shakespeare recognised, speaking through Edgar in Act IV of *King Lear*: "the worst is not/ So long as we can say 'This is the worst'." Something "unbearable" can still be borne—that is its deeper meaning.

"Inconsolable" is another word that doesn't mean exactly what it says. The seemingly irremediable hurt that made you describe yourself as such is also a request for solace. My hand on your shoulder is an expression of sympathy for the ineffability of your experience, as well as an acknowledgement that your personal sorrow, translated, is also the collective human one.

Tact

It is one of those qualities which render modern life bearable. Tact, from the Latin *tactus*, had long existed as a cognate for the faculty of touch, and is preserved in English in the adjectives *tactile* and, more remotely, *tangible*. Some historians have interpreted the famous voice (or *daimon*) that Socrates listened out for as a kind of "spiritual tact" preventing him from acting in any way detrimental to his true interests. But tact, as "a ready and delicate sense of what is fitting and proper in dealing with others, so as to avoid giving offence or to win good will", appeared, according to the OED, only in 1804, at the beginning of the century that would see the Industrial Revolution give rise to increasing urbanisation, social mobility and alienation between persons.

Tact was the new code of discretion that appeared when absolutism lost its head, and the middle classes began to dominate the political and economic scene with notions of "fellow-feeling" or "sympathy". It took over from the conventional polite behaviour and courtly manner expected of the gentry even as courtesy—like aristocratic *tenue* itself—still survives. It is the one virtue that might be thought to possess purely formal qualities. Even Nietzsche saw courtesy as an important convention: rudeness (blunt German rudeness) betrayed a fundamental flaw—a lack of style and self-discipline. "Where a human being finds himself in such proximity to human beings," wrote Robert Walser in his 1907 prose piece "Friedrichstrasse", about one of the busiest streets in Berlin, "the concept *neighbour* takes on a genuinely practical, comprehensible, and swiftly grasped meaning." After all, tact has a musical sense too.

With the rise of mercantile life came the realisation that we are apt to tread on other people's toes and unwittingly inflict all kinds of upset. (*The public*, after all, is as much an invention of nineteenth-century gentility as tact.) For if modern emotional life seems to be dominated by jealousy, envy and greed, it is not so much because these temperaments have mysteriously increased (though it would be odd if a society which is constructed on the illusion of the fully informed, rational and self-interested economic actor didn't—against its own better intentions—*encourage* them), but because other people are both necessary to our getting what we want, and obstacles to it too. With the beginning of modernity came the end of spontaneity: there was no longer a straight line between the subject and the object of his desire. All sorts of things and people get in the way of our getting on. These negative emotions are what Stendhal called *vanité*: aping and imitating other people who are essentially our equals and whom we endow with a largely arbitrary prestige. Self-centredness is agonisingly other-centredness too. Socially, we are hypocrites, and obliged to be.

This is the sore point. Without common agreements and settlements, we have no means of measuring tact. As individuals become emancipated from even minimal inherited conventions, exercising old-fashioned tact can often seem to be inquisitive or prying—"What business is it of yours anyway?"—or craven, as in the old British habit of apologising in advance. "Why should you be sorry?" Tact can even come to seem like tactlessness—a parody of itself. The outcome is antagonism. As Adorno says, "To write off convention as an outdated, useless and extraneous ornament is only to confirm the most extraneous of all things, a life of direct domination." The only place left for tact to go, among the solitudes of modern life, is back to its physical origins.

My traditional sense of tact has compelled me to stop doctoring. My (critical) tactlessness is to keep writing.

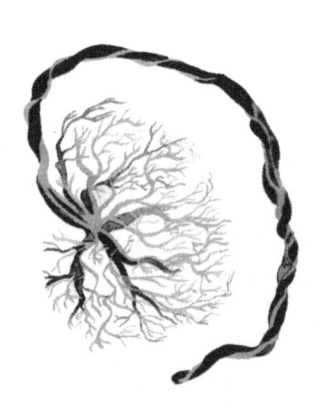

Acknowledgements

For many years I had wanted to write a kind of commonplace book of my own experience inside and out of the medical profession, an account both encyclopaedic and personal that would break the crust of convention, but hardly knew how to begin. "You're going to have to go beyond the clinical…", W. H. Auden advised Oliver Sacks after he published his first book. "Be metaphorical, be mystical, be whatever you need". Solid advice for any "medical" writer. But it was only when I serendipitously discovered a book called *The Silence of the Body* in English translation on the shelves of a London bookshop that I saw a way into the present work. That was well over twenty years ago.

The Silence of the Body (1979) is one of the many publications of the prolific Bible scholar, essayist and puppetmaster Guido Ceronetti: it was an unlikely bestseller in the original Italian and remains his only work to have been translated into English. When it appeared in translation, one medical reviewer found it too provocative and strange, too "weird" for him to make much sense of it. (Never be afraid of your little bit of weirdness, confides the Swiss German writer Robert Walser.) It was precisely the baroque aspects of Ceronetti's scrapbook, written over many years too, that appealed to me, even if I felt compelled to argue with some of his assertions (he is on firm ground with semitic nounforms, less so with contemporary science). His fragments lend a depth to medicine, although it is a depth that medicine has shed in its modern transformation into a technical discipline. I wasn't taught any medical history at my medical school in Glasgow: almost everywhere the field is regarded as a subdiscipline of the arts faculty rather than an adjunct of medicine itself. And there are good reasons for that, aside from an already crowded curriculum. Medicine is a profession in which what used to be called "common sense" has a high standing: too big a serving of its often richly embarrassing history would be to tip it into the opposite mode of irony. An ironist (as Richard Rorty tells us) is someone who has doubts about his own final vocabulary, his place in life and even his moral identity—all considerations that are very far from the minds of people who never think twice about the vocabulary they employ. Doctors are professionals whose commitment to the real holds them back from self-knowledge.

When Ceronetti asserts, in the introduction to his book, that "Medicine is a philosophical discipline that can be studied in any number of ways, going to medical school among them", he is being anachronistic. For sure, back in 1696, the great German philosopher Gottfried Leibniz could write to his French correspondent Guillaume François de l'Hospital: "May it please God that it should come about that doctors philosophise, and philosophers occupy themselves with medicine." Doctors now rarely philosophise (or even have the time to do so), but at one time medicine and philosophy were inseparable: the great second-century Roman physician Galen wrote a tract entitled "That the Best Physician is also a Philosopher". Ceronetti, a touch immodestly, sees himself as one of these philosophising physicians in search of the truth, and justifies himself thus: "for the truth is always therapeutic, masterfully surgical, and splendidly philanthropic."

The "scattered limbs" of my title perhaps conjure up an unappealingly mangled prospect—something like Géricault's 1820 study of amputated limbs, done after visits to the morgue of the Hôpital Beaujon in Paris. For all its horrific subject matter, Géricault's treatment of distressed body parts exerts a kind of fascination: his depiction of them is almost tender. In fact, my concern in writing these entries has throughout been more anthropological than anatomical (although I can see an unexpected link between Géricault and the Dada artist Hannah Höch, whose series *Aus einem ethnographischen Museum* (1924–30) makes an audacious attempt to represent the "living collages" of soldiers patched up after the First World War); and I also sought a link to the classical world—the great discovery of my early years in education. "Scattered limbs" echoes the Latin phrase "disiecta membra" ("scattered fragments"), used to refer to surviving bits or shards of ancient manuscripts and other cultural objects. It derives from a line in a poem by the Latin poet Horace, "disiecti membra poetae", which is taken to imply that even if lines from a poet's work are dispersed or disaggregated (like Humpty Dumpty), they will still be recognisably *his*.

Calling a book *Scattered Limbs* is a risky strategy, especially a book that seeks to understand medicine in the round; when I had assembled most of my entries, my working title still seemed a fitting one—I had been won over by the formulaic brevity of the fragment. The title further commended itself to me by echoing J. P. Stern's *A Doctrine of Scattered Occasions*, a fine textual study of one of my cultural heroes Georg Christoph Lichtenberg (1742–99), natural scientist, Göttingen professor and unabashed Anglophile, whose most celebrated work in his lifetime was a study of Hogarth. Lichtenberg is famous for his *Sudelbücher* or "wastebooks": these were jotters to which he committed his brilliantly witty observations on all kinds of topics, from the novel smallpox vaccine to the revolution taking place in France. His "occasions" of thinking for himself fill 900 pages in my German edition of his work and are considered one of that language's greatest stylistic achievements.

Then there's the subtitle. Why call it a "dreambook" when there aren't that many dreams in it? As it must have seemed to Hannah Höch and those madcap surrealists of the 1930s, medicine's own repressed history offers traction for the imagination: there may be only one or two actual dreams in *Scattered Limbs*, but the entire book is a kind of dream-incubator. It dreams in the broadest sense. After all, magico-mechanical elements have their place in all ritual effects, and techniques were being "dreamed up" long before they become labour-saving shortcuts. Henri Ellenberger's *The Discovery of the Unconscious* (1970) begins with the animal magnetism of Mesmer at the end of the eighteenth century, and grinds to a halt in 1945, when collective irrationality almost conquered the world: war's end is conventionally figured as the advent of the Leviathan-like health systems that cocoon us today.

I also found theoretical justification for my approach where I hadn't expected to find it: in a short appreciation of the work of the surrealist artist Max Ernst by Claude Lévi-Strauss ("Une peinture méditative", in *Un Regard Éloigné*, 1983). Recollecting that Ernst had referred to the famous "chance encounter on a dissection table of a sewing machine and an umbrella"—an episode in Lautréamont's proto-surrealist text *Les Chants de*

Maldoror (1859)—as an illustration of his artistic method, the anthropologist suggested that his work on the structure of myths had developed in a manner analogous to that of the painter. He had come upon them in the field as so many images found at random in old books, cropped them and allowed them to rearrange themselves, not consciously and deliberately, but following their own orderings and promptings in his mind. We are being asked to believe that what the surrealists were to painting, Lévi-Strauss is to anthropology.

Not such a *chance* encounter then. It is an unexpected revelation by the great structuralist. I hope that it was not presumptuous to take this primal coupling as a model for my own operating procedure.

*

Some of these entries in this book first appeared elsewhere, and I would like to thank the editors of the following journals for allowing me to republish and sometimes develop earlier versions: *British Journal of General Practice* (London) which included an illustrated series as its Christmas special in 2008, *Quadrant* (Sydney) which ran a sequence under the title "My Hand is my Heart", *PN Review* (Manchester) for scattered items in my column "Catchwords" (2009–16) and the bilingual publication *Klasik nan Asyik* (Jakarta), a product of the Utan Kayu Salahari Literary Biennale 2011; the entry on the poet and dermatologist Gottfried Benn was first published as a letter to the *London Review of Books*.

Friends and correspondents have discussed entries with me, and on some occasions made helpful suggestions: I would like to thank in particular Les Murray, Frederic Raphael, Douglas Shenson, John and Mary Gillies, Brian Hurwitz, Neil Vickers, Michael Schmidt, Bruce Charlton, Gerald Mangan, Desmond Avery, Peter and Maria McCarey, Christine and Richard Thayer, Raymond Bach, Gregory Owcarz, Jeremy Garwood and two stalwart medical colleagues in Paris, Olivier Wong and Frank Slattery. Suggestions in letters from Jeff Aronson and Richard Lehmann were also helpful. All the opinions expressed in this book should of course be regarded as my own attempts to get a grip on things. Long ago, my classics teacher at school in Glasgow, Mr (Duncan) Sinclair, primed me by setting Plato's *Phaedo* as reading material: why the dying Socrates should instruct his friend Crito "to offer a cock to Asclepius" is still a puzzle, perhaps even a scandal, to interpreters. The philosopher's parody of the convalescent's usual act of thanks to the god of healing strikes me now as being a bit like our old family GP, Dr Kelly, *instructing* me as a wide-eyed young boy to be cheeky: Stick out your tongue! So I did. A routine medical act had a hidden meaning. I was getting nearer the heart of the mystery.

It has become customary to be pious about medicine, but I have strong misgivings about piety (having been brought up in an atmosphere of the willed kind): laughter is more honest, and comes from the intestines, as the great French writer (and doctor) Rabelais knew. Over the years I've learned to live in different cultures, and to let those voices guide me. On convivial occasions with my father-in-law Christian Schütze, I profited from his knowledge of the German classics, recited from memory, as well as his experience as home affairs editor for the *Süddeutsche Zeitung*; my wife and I attended to him in his last days in February 2018, providing an extended palliative "house call". My daughter Claire supplied the book's opening and closing illustrations, and my son Felix has helped to develop my website, part of which is given over to my medical writings (and where the reader can find a list of works cited in the individual sections of *Scattered Limbs*). My persevering wife Cornelia has kept me in touch with the impact of TQM (total quality management) on the nursing profession on both sides of the Rhine. Thanks are also due to Robert Hyde at Galileo, who saw potential in the book from the very first.

Although it was Richard Rorty who best defined the contemporary ironist (*supra*), it was a reading of Alasdair MacIntyre's *After Virtue* that convinced me to abandon my attempt to freight my skills to Strasbourg, obliging me to realise that I couldn't flourish as a medical practitioner under the conditions that apply to medical practice in France. This reversal of circumstances is no argument against France, but it fingers—at least to my mind—what Larry Siedentop has identified as the "almost primitive simplicity" of the British constitution and the inability of its political class to make a constructive contribution to Europe. If the United Kingdom has been unable to export its social self-understanding to Europe it is because the country has never had to be explicit about its arrangements for living. Manners are still what count, not ideas.

★

These notes have been completed in the week in which Britain—the country which first came up with representative government, the form of government adopted by much of the world—formally left the European Union. Voltaire is perhaps the best known of the many commentators who sometimes grudgingly, sometimes enthusiastically looked on the parliament in London as something of a marvel, and certainly worth emulating: it was a beacon of hope for liberal ambitions. It is therefore with some trepidation that I watch my native country take a leap into the dark. I did that once myself, attempting to see what substance there was in Council Directive 93/16/EEC of 5 April 1993 on the free movement of doctors and recognition of their formal qualifications in the European Union. In hindsight a mistake, but without its lessons this book would not have been written.

So here we are. Disjected, but not wholly dejected.

Strasbourg, 31 January 2020